EMERGING INFECTIOUS DISEASES IN INDIA

EMERGING INFECTIOUS DISEASES IN INDIA

VIROJ WIWANITKIT
AND
MOHEN Y. SINGH

Nova Biomedical Books
New York

For permission to use material from this book please contact us:
Telephone 631-231-7269; Fax 631-231-8175
Web Site: http://www.novapublishers.com

Library of Congress Cataloging-in-Publication Data

Viroj Wiwanitkit.
Emerging infectious diseases in india / Viroj Wiwanitkit and Mohen Y. Singh.
p. ; cm.
Includes bibliographical references and index.
ISBN 978-1-60741-168-0 (hardcover)
1. Emerging infectious diseases--India. I. Singh, Mohen Y. II. Title.
[DNLM: 1. Communicable Diseases, Emerging--epidemiology--India. 2. Communicable Diseases, Emerging--prevention & control--India. 3. Communicable Disease Control--organization & administration--India. 4. Developing Countries--India. WA 110 V819e 2009]
RA643.I4V57 2009
362.196'90954--dc22 2009003887

Published by Nova Science Publishers, Inc. ✢ New York

Contents

Preface

Human immunodeficiency virus or HIV infection is a very well known viral infection in the present day. This is defined as a new emerging viral infection in the past 2 decades. At this time, this is not an emerging infection. However, it is associated with other relating emerging infections. Those infections are due to the immunodeficiency stage in the HIV infected cases. At the time of discovery, the impaired immune status is the presentation of affected cases. This is a mysterious for a long time. After the succeed in identification of HIV virus, this disease became well known and accepted as the most important immunodeficiency syndrome. HIV is accepted as the pathogenic organism. Indeed, HIV infection seems to be a complex disease. There are many researches and developments for HIV. There is also specific branch of medicine called HIV medicine. The knowledge on HIV infection is required for all physicians at present.

Chapter I - India is a very famous country in Asia. However, in another sense, India means a subcontinent of Asia, which is previously called Pink Continent or "Chompootaveep." This area covers many countries that combine South Asia. These countries are India, Bangladesh, Pakistan, Bhutan, Nepal, Sri-lanka and Maldives. This specific area has a very old history. Thousands years before, human beings lived here and created many specific culture of India, which is presently well known. This is considered as a world's oldest culture. Culture and society of India is very specific and this brings the well known Indian style. Considering the location of India, it lies between two important parts of the world, the Middle East, the world of Islamic culture, and the East as well as Southeast Asia, another world's heritage area. This makes India as a gate between several cultures for years. For sure, this affects lifestyle of the Indian and it can have several effects on health.

Chapter II - Leptospirosis is an important spirochete infection. The pathogenic organism is a spiral or helical shaped prokaryote and is an obligate aerobe that is highly motile. Concerning the natural history of this infection, the pathogenic organism which is excreted in urine by rats and other infected mammals can be transmitted in contaminated water, usually flood water. The infected person gets the germ by direct contact with a skin wound, especially at the foot. Not wearing shoes and walking in flood water is a risk-filled behavior for this infection. Leptospirosis is an important tropical disease with high prevalence in many tropical countries. Presenting symptoms vary with age: children showing primarily fever, vomiting, headache, abdominal and generalized muscle pain and diarrhea while adults usually have fever, headache, anorexia, myalgia and constipation. However, fever is the main symptom and can be misdiagnosed with other common tropical infections which usually present with fever. Myalgia, especially at the calf, is also common. Also, this can be mimicked by other common tropical infections.

Chapter III - Malaria is an important tropical mosquito-borne protozoa infection. It can be noted that malaria is a very important tropical mosquito-borne infectious disease affecting millions of the world's population annually. Malaria is caused by specific parasites of the genus Plasmodium. Five species of *Plasmodium*, *Plasmodium falciparum*, *Plasmodium vivax*, *Plasmodium ovale*, *Plasmodium malariae* and *Plasmodium knowlesii* can produce the human disease in its several forms. In humans, malaria is a potentially deadly mosquito-borne disease characterized by cyclical patterns of fever with severe myalgia, shaking and sweating found in the tropical countries. Despite encouraging trends of decreasing malaria, the rates of the disease may be re-emerging in many tropical and non-tropical countries, especially in Asia, as evidence from an increased annual parasite index. Despite several years of malarial control success and a competent network of countrywide health infrastructure, malaria is still an important health threat in rural communities at present. Members of 5 anopheline species complexes, *Anopheles dirus*, *Anopheles minimus*, *Anopheles sandicus*, *Anopheles aconitus* and *Anopheles manculatus*, registered to be primary malaria vectors, are also common in many tropical countries.

Chapter IV - Leishmaniasis is an important tropical vector-borne infection. There are two main forms of leishmaniasis, the cutaneous and visceral forms. Leishmanioses are a group of blood parasitic diseases that affect man and also other mammals. The infections are caused by different species of trypanosomatids of the genus Leishmania. Leishmaniasis is confirmed as a complex of diseases with a clinical and epidemiological diversity. Leishmaniasis is still a severe public health problem and its burden is increasing in many countries. As already mentioned, this disease is generated by a parasite belonging to the genus Leishmania. Approximately 350 billion people in 88 different countries are noted to be infected with this parasite. The distribution of this re-emerging disease, which is found throughout the world, is believed to be due to various factors linked to both human activity and climatic change. The heteroecious life cycle of this blood parasite includes an invertebrate host (sandflies of the Phlebotomidae family). The dog is the main carrier of this disease.

Chapter V - Dengue infection is a mosquito-borne arboviral infectious disease. The infection of the virus brings a variable spectrum of the illness that runs from a simple fever to severe dengue hemorrhagic fever (HDF), a fatal disease. Mairuhu et al said that dengue fever came to be more recognized as one of the greater contagious illnesses owing to increased incident and spreading geographical distribution of dengue fever in the past years. Nogueira said that dengue fever was one of the very frequent predominant acute fevers and might be extremely fatal if associated with complications. Halstead said that the antibodies played significant roles in protecting and expanding infections of dengue fever, therefore, there are ongoing studies trying to find the final knowledge of what parts in the human body are infected by the human dengue fever and trying to gain a comprehension of early antibody-accessible steps of the infection concentrating on cellular level. Nogueira also noted that control of vector was still the most effective means of preventive medicine. There have been many efforts in the last six decades to produce a vaccine to fight this infection. According to globalization in the present, the dengue fever shows arising patterns not only tropical but also in non-tropical countries. Wilson recently said that travelers could also be seen as carriers that harbor pathogen and microbial genetic matter to other regions of the world where investigators could carry out detailed analyses that could help map the location and movement of strains, genotypes and resistance patterns. The knowledge about dengue infection is, therefore, an interesting theme for general physicians around the world.

Chapter VI - Chikungunya fever is a viral infection generating hemorrhagic fever similar to the dengue virus infection. Chikungunya virus is noted as an arbovirus in group A.

It is classified as a virus in the family Togaviridae. Chikungunya fever is a viral disease transmitted to human beings by Aedes genus mosquitoes. The chikungunya virus is highly infective and its incubation period is 3-12 days. With regard to the clinical manifestations, sudden severe headache, the colds, fever, joint pain and myalgia are the most common symptoms. Children can also show additional neurological symptoms. The hemorrhagic fever is a serious complication of this infection; however, the hemorrhage is not common and can recede in 3-5 days. Antigens or antibody study is the main diagnosis for this infection. An IgM ELISA is necessary to make differential diagnoses of dengue fever. The application of the molecular diagnosis of the infection of Chikungunya virus has also been noted in medicine for the past few years. The acute hemorrhagic fever of caused by Chikungunya infection can be managed with the similar protocols to dengue fever.

Chapter VII - Japanese encephalitis is another mosquito-borne arboviral infection. Globally, the Japanese encephalitis virus is arising as a more important viral encephalitis despite the vaccine being available. Solomon said that recent work on the Japanese encephalitis virus suggested that the virus has its origin in the specific area of Indonesian-Malaya, and in some extending areas. For a few years, significant advances have been made due to the understanding of natural history and pathogenesis of this deadly mosquito borne viral encephalitis. Mackenzie et al noted that mosquito-borne flaviviruses inclusive Japanese encephalitis virus provided some of the most important examples to arise on resurging infections of global significance. Gubler said that there had been a resurgence or dramatic increase of illnesses of arboviral or epidemic including Japanese encephalitis, affecting both humans and pets. Zeller said that the air transportation permitted the fast changing site from place to place as well as the diffusion of potential vectors and infected host.

Chapter VIII - India is a developing country in Asia with high prevalence of gastrointestinal infection. As already mentioned in the first chapter, India can also be expressed as a subcontinent of Asia covering many countries that combine to form South Asia. Many specific cultures of India, which are presently well known, exist. This is considered to be the world's oldest rooted culture which affects the lifestyle of the Indian and has several effects on health. Due to the highly populated characteristics, India has many public health problems. This is the common cause of communicable disease in India. For sure, these gastrointestinal infectious diseases can cause very high mortality and morbidity. Also, there are many emerging and reemerging gastrointestinal infectious diseases in India. The specific aim of this chapter is to focus on those emerging and reemerging gastrointestinal infectious diseases in India.

Chapter IX - Hepatitis by definition is the inflammation of the hepatic cell. There are many possible causes of hepatitis in medicine. These can be infectious or non-infectious. The hepatitis virus can be seen elsewhere around the world. However, high prevalence of hepatitis can be seen in the tropical regions. This might be due to the high rate of infectious hepatitis cases in this area. Concerning the signs and symptoms of hepatitis, the common presentation is jaundice, which implies disturbance of the bile system. Jaundice can be easily divided by its etiology as pre-hepatic, hepatic and post-hepatic types. However, jaundice does not mean injury or inflammation of hepatic cells. The direct reflection of the hepatic cell problem is the increased level of the hepatic enzyme. In laboratory medicine, the common liver function tests that imply the hepatic cellular condition are the two enzymes named SGOT and SGPT. These two enzymes are usually the basic diagnostic tools for hepatitis. The other hepatic profiles are not directly related to hepatic cellular disorder. Increased amounts of transaminase enzymes can be the clue for diagnosis of hepatitis. The other presentations of hepatitis include fever, fatigue, abdominal pain and myalgia, which are all weak signs and symptoms.

The term tropical hepatitis in this chapter means the condition of hepatitis that is specific to the nature of tropical countries. This can be either infection or non-infection related. Examples of infectious tropical hepatitis are several kinds of viral hepatitis diseases. Examples of non-infectious tropical hepatitis are several kinds of intoxications. When we talk about tropical hepatitis, ones usually tends to focus on the infection. Indeed, infection is a common problem in tropical countries and many infections can lead to the problem of hepatitis. The most common infectious disorder that brings tropical hepatitis is viral hepatitis. Viral hepatitis means the specific kind of hepatitis that is caused by the hepatitis virus. Hepatitis virus by definition means a group of viruses that can cause hepatitis in infected subjects. There are many kinds of hepatitis viruses that are still problematic around the world. There are several means of transmission. Details of each important hepatitis virus will be further discussed in this chapter.

Chapter X - Tuberculosis is one of the most important infectious diseases in the world. On average, one-third of the world's population is expected to get this infection. There are millions of people who get new infections annually. There are also millions of deaths due to tuberculosis every year. The diagnosis and treatment of tuberculosis are known by physicians around the world. The common clinical presentation of tuberculosis include the chronic cough (for more than 3 months), hemoptysis, low grade fever, fatigue, night sweating, as well as weight loss. However, these symptoms are not specific. There are also many other tropical infections that can provide similar symptoms.

Chapter XI - Anal tuberculosis is not an uncommon pathology found in the tropics. A tuberculous origin must be considered when the cause of perianal lesion is unclear to avoid undesirable delay in the diagnosis and treatment of this disease. This brief treatise explores the different etiopathogenic, clinical, and diagnostic manifestations of ano-perianal tuberculosis.

Chapter XII - From time immemorial, the two mycobacterial diseases tuberculosis and leprosy have ranked amongst the most feared and dreaded diseases that afflict mankind. The genus Mycobacterium is responsible for more misery and suffering than any other genus of bacteria. Tuberculosis was dubbed by the evangelist John Bunyan as "the captain of all these men of death". It was also known as "Rajayakshma", which means 'the king of diseases', while leprosy, caused by *Mycobacterium leprae* is termed the 'disease of kings'.

With the introduction of many public health measures and chemotherapy during the second half of this century, there was a dramatic decline in the morbidity and mortality, due to tuberculosis. .

However, tuberculosis actually is on the rise again, especially among the homeless, alcohol and drug abuse population and the AIDS patients. The increasing number of multi-drug resistant strains of *Mycobacterium tuberculosis* isolates from both AIDS and non-AIDS patients is an ominous trend that threatens tuberculosis eradication programmes worldwide.

Chapter XIII - Suppurative pathologies associated with chronic anal fissures are common but are not well documented. Fissure abscess, post fissure fistula, and post fissure antibioma are but a few of them. These pathologies increase the complications and morbidity of the primary lesion and need a comprehensive approach. From the hospital case record of 532 patients treated for chronic anal fissures, 88 (16.5%) were found to have one of these pathologies. This retrospective study describes such pathologies in terms of demographics, clinical presentation, pathological features, operative technique and the outcome. 95% of the patients presented with pain and discharge per anus. Following the surgical procedure, 90% of them could resume their duties within a week. Wound healing took a period between 2 weeks to 2 months. At the last follow up at 18 months, three patients had a recurrence (3.4%). Suppuration in chronic anal fissure seems to be more frequent than described. While dealing with the anal fissure, it is desirable to look for these associated pathologies as well to avoid complications and morbidity of the primary disease.

Chapter XIV - Bird flu or atypical avian influenza is kind of influenza. The bird flu virus can cause the respiratory tract infection owing to the nature of general influenza. Basically, influenza virus can be classified into 3 groups: A, B and C. The classification relies mainly on the difference of nucleoprotein and matrix antigens. In addition, influenza can also be divided into subtypes depending on hosts. Influenza viruses have their spherical shape with average size about 1000 A in diameter and have an as yet undefined central structure containing the eight negative-sense RNA particles of the genome in association with the transcriptase required for mRNA synthesis, an abundant nucleoprotein, and a similarly abundant matrix protein. This core is surrounded by a membrane got from the cell surface in a budding process by which newly formed viruses are secreted out from the infected cell. During infection cell membranes are affected by the incorporation of newly synthesized virus membrane proteins. As a result, the released viruses contain exclusively two different kinds of virus-specified glycoprotein, hemagglutinin and neuraminidase, and a proton channel protein, M2. As previously mentioned, the influenza viruses have segmented, negative stranded RNA genomes (vRNA) and are also enveloped. The viruses can be derived from the plasma membrane of many cells especially for the apical plasma membrane of polarized epithelial cells. Complete virus particles are not found inside infected cells. Virus particles is composed of three major subviral components, namely the viral envelope, matrix protein (M1), and core (viral ribonucleocapsid [vRNP]). Several kinds of interactions that lead to virus assembly are described, including interactions between matrix proteins and membranes, interactions between matrix proteins and glycoproteins, interactions between matrix proteins and nucleocapsids, as well as interactions that lead to matrix protein self-assembly. For viral morphogenesis to occur, all three viral components, namely the viral envelope, M1, and the vRNP have to be led to the assembly site at previously mentioned cells. Finally, buds need to be created at the assembly site and virus particles released with the closure of buds. These are important basic knowledge in virology of influenza virus.

Chapter XV - Scrub typhus by definition is an infection caused by rickettsial pathogen, *Orientia tsutsugamushi*. The pathogen, an obligate intracellular bacterium, was firstly isolated in 1930. There are many possible infections due to rickettsia in medicine. The rickettsial infection can be seen elsewhere around the world. However, scrub typhus is the rickettsial infection that is common in the tropical regions. This might be due to the nature of the pathogen and the abundance of insect vector in this area. Scrub typhus is a vector borne disease. The tick is the vector for this infection. Scrub typhus is endemic in Asia. Local people's behavior and climatic changes can influence the occurrence of the disease. Concerning the nature of vector borne disease, it relates strongly to the poverty as well as climate. Poverty means poor and this prevents good sanitation. Insect vector is more prevalent in the places with poor sanitation. This is also the places for the poor. India has millions of the poor, therefore, abundance of vectors can be expected. Focusing on the climate, the hot monsoon type climate helps propagate of the insect vector and this is the actual climate of the tropical countries of Asia. Increasing prevalences of scrub typhus have been reported from some Asian countries and may accompany with the widespread use of beta-lactam antibiotics or to improve diagnostic tools.

Chapter XVI - Mainly, outbreaks of buffalopox affect buffaloes, cows and humans in many parts of the world. Since the first outbreak in India, a large number of epidemics are reported around the world. This affects the dairy industry. Singh et al reported that the causative pathogen, buffalopox virus (BPXV), was a member of the Orthopoxvirus, and was closely related to Vaccinia virus (VACV), the type-species of the genus. Tuner and Baxby observed that controlled degradation of virions showed that the polypeptides which enabled the viruses to be differentiated were located in the surface and sub-surface layers. Tuner and Baxby noted that this might relate to the infectious property. *Dumbell* and *Richardson* performed virological investigations of specimens from buffaloes affected by buffalopox in Maharashtra State, India between 1985 and 1987. In this work, isolates of poxviruses were made from specimens of scabs taken from pox lesions on buff. *Dumbell* and *Richardson* found that the biological characters of most isolates resembled those of the Hissar strain of buffalopox virus, except for one isolate which appeared to be vaccinia. They finally concluded that buffalopox was an emerging enzootic virus and was a subspecies of vaccinia virus. Until present, continuous researches on this new emerging viruses are still undergone.

Chapter XVII - Human immunodeficiency virus or HIV infection is a very well known viral infection in the present day. This is defined as a new emerging viral infection in the past 2 decades. At this time, this is not an emerging infection. However, it is associated with other relating emerging infections. Those infections are due to the immunodeficiency stage in the HIV infected cases. At the time of discovery, the impaired immune status is the presentation of affected cases. This is a mysterious for a long time. After the succeed in identification of HIV virus, this disease became well known and accepted as the most important immunodeficiency syndrome. HIV is accepted as the pathogenic organism. Indeed, HIV infection seems to be a complex disease. There are many researches and developments for HIV. There is also specific branch of medicine called HIV medicine. The knowledge on HIV infection is required for all physicians at present

Chapter I

India: A Model for Health in Developing World

Where is India?

India is a very famous country in Asia. However, in another sense, India means a subcontinent of Asia, which is previously called Pink Continent or "Chompootaveep." This area covers many countries that combine South Asia. These countries are India, Bangladesh, Pakistan, Bhutan, Nepal, Sri-lanka and Maldives. This specific area has a very old history. Thousands years before, human beings lived here and created many specific culture of India, which is presently well known. This is considered as a world's oldest culture. Culture and society of India is very specific and this brings the well known Indian style. Considering the location of India, it lies between two important parts of the world, the Middle East, the world of Islamic culture, and the East as well as Southeast Asia, another world's heritage area. This makes India as a gate between several cultures for years. For sure, this affects lifestyle of the Indian and it can have several effects on health.

Health in India [1 - 6]

At present, millions of people live in India. India is one of the heavy populated areas in the world. Due to the high populated characteristics, India faces up with challenge in public health. It can be said that India has several public health problems, similar to other Asian developing countries, and this leads us to specific concern on India. Although present India has many advanced technology in many big cities the other rooted behaviors and poor sanitation can also be seen in many poor rural area of the country. How to manage the health problem within India is of interest. As a summary to the reader, the author will hereby summarize and present the core problem in health within India.

1. Communicable disease

   Communicable diseases are common in India. There are many infectious diseases reported in India. Due to the nature of developing counties, many infectious diseases are still problematic. For sure, these infectious diseases cause very high mortality and morbidity. Also, there are many emerging and remerging diseases in India. The specific aim of this book is to focus on those emerging and remerging infectious disease in India.

2. Non communicable disease

   Similar to communicable disease, due to the nature of developing country, several non communicable diseases are reported from India annually. These include intoxication, accident and metabolic disorders. Crowded populations are being high risk for many problems in India. How to manage these problematic situations is a challenge to the local public health care workers.

It is clear that the problem exists. The other additional thought is on what the etiology of those described conditions is. Indeed, this can be easily talked. There are surely several preventable and non preventable underlying factors for the problematic conditions. The author will hereby present the details of these factors.

1. Inherited factor

For sure, inherited factor or genetic factor can contribute to several kinds of medical disorders. It should be noted that there are some specific disorders that are common or specific in India. Hemoglobinopathy is a well described genetic disorder. Hemoglobin Q India is the best example of specific hemoglobinopathy reported from India. Hemoglobin Q-India is an endemic hemoglobinopathy in India that was first identified in India. Hb Q-India is caused by the mutation from the specific sequence GAC to CAC at codon 64 of the alpha-1 globin gene. The correlation between this hemoglobinopathy and thalassemia was well reported. Wiwanitkit found that the main difference between the predicted alpha globin secondary structures of normal and Hb Q-India is an extra helix in the Hb Q-India. The predicted tertiary structure also supports this finding [7].

2. Non inherited factor

Non inherited facto or environmental factor is very important. There are many non inherited factors that affect the health status of the Indian. Of these factors, poverty and sanitation should be mentioned. There are many reports from India on the effect of poverty on the health status of the Indian. These interesting reports will be briefly presented in Table 1.

Table 1. Some interesting reports on effect of poverty on health status of the Indian.

Authors	Details
Muniyandi and Ramachandran [8]	Muniyandi and Ramachandran studied on Socioeconomic inequalities of tuberculosis in India [8]. They reported that poverty was the main determinant for inequalities of tuberculosis [8].
Ramaraj and Alpert [9]	Ramaraj and Alpert studied on Indian poverty and cardiovascular disease [9]. They said that "There is a clear progression to degenerative and lifestyle-related diseases such as cardiovascular disease as a result of current social and economic change.[9]" Finally, Ramaraj and Alpert addressed the imminent threats and ways to tackle the epidemic in India [9].
Dror et al [10]	Dror et al summarized that "Interventions to reduce the cost of illness should be context-specific, as there is no "one-size-fits-all" model to establish the cost of healthcare for the entire India.[10]." Dror et al noted that aggregated expenses might cause catastrophic consequences of medical disorder [10].
Kumar et al [11]	Kumar et al studied on gap between awareness and practices regarding maternal and child health among women in an urban slum community in India [11]. Kumar et al suggested for the requirement for bridging the existing gaps avoiding socio-cultural barriers and misconceptions prevailing in the community and by promoting and protecting healthy maternal and child care practices [11].
Bose et al [12]	Bose et al reported on high levels of underweight and stunting among pre-adolescent children of low socioeconomic class from Madhyamgram and Barasat, West Bengal, India [12].
McDermott et al [13]	McDermott et al said that identified barriers to the development of palliative care in India included: poverty, population density, geography, opioid availability, workforce development, and limited national palliative care policy. [13].
Srivastava et al [14]	Srivastava et al studied on Neonatal morbidity and care-seeking behavior in urban Lucknow, India [14]. They noted that severe neonatal illnesses were proved significantly higher among neonates from slums as compared to those from non-slum areas [14].

Some Social Backgrounds of India

Before we jump into the further topics on this book, it is necessary to know the history of India. Some social backgrounds of India have to be mentioned. India is one of the oldest site of the world. The history of India rolled back for thousands of years. There are many dynasties in Indian history before India becomes present republic state. Of interest, several religions including Hinduism, Buddhism and Sikha have its originality in India. Presently, those religions still exist. There are also external religions that are presently believed and practiced in India including Christian and Islam. The rooted cultures based on these described religions still exist. The social background of India is very complex. The rooted culture of Hinduism, the major religion of the Indian, affects a lot. There are many rooted traditions resulted from Hinduism. These Hinduism based traditions sometimes affect health status of the Indian population. Some specific groups of Indian populations are very poor and far from good health service. Moreover, some are very rich and lived in well conditioned buildings. These can highly consume the heath service facilities. In addition, although there are many people in Indian, they are not united but classified by their birth status due to rooted Hinduism belief. India is a country considered very crowded comparing to the limited area. Discrepancy between the Indian can be seen. Also, several rooted cultured bound and religious based behaviors bring risks to the populations who practice those behaviors.

The next step is to clarify the effect of complex social background on health status of the Indian. Indeed, this is already mentioned as this is the fact of non inherited factor. Poverty is the main factor contributing to poor health status. Indeed, poverty means no money in its easy way. Therefore, poor Indian cannot afford the cost for their health facilities. How to get rid of the poverty in India is the main question because the poverty in India is the big problem. However, this dose not imply that the rich in India have to have no risk. Some rooted culture bounded believes in India also contribute to high risk for poor health status.

At the present day, the concept of social medicine is emerging because it cannot be avoided that social backgrounds have a lot of impacts on health status. The approach of social medicine act to cope with the health problem in India is feasible. To help the reader better understand on the concept, the author hereby will present case studies as demo.

The first case is a university teacher who has a disability on her left leg due to the poliomyelitis complication in her younger lifetime. She usually visited to the rural area for researching and teaching. She got a high fever for a month but she prescribed herself for some drugs. She is a medical scientist and believed on her pharmaceutical knowledge. However, the symptoms were not improved. Finally, she went to the physician and finally found to have malaria. This case is delayed for diagnosis and treatment. The good social backgrounds of this patient do not help early diagnosis. Perhaps, this case has a long termed disability and makes the patient to tolerate to any suffering. In addition, due to the high education, the patient tried to prescribe the drug for herself instead of visiting to the physician to get the correct diagnosis.

The second scenario is the case of a Buddhist monk who lived in the forest. He is not poor but practices due to the specific principles of Buddhism that is called Tudongavatara. This principle indicates living to practice within the deep forest. He had high fever for months but not visited to any physician. Finally, his pupils felt that this was not acceptable therefore they brought this monk to the physician. This monk was finally diagnosed to have vivax malaria. This case is another good example. The delay of diagnosis in this case is not due to the poverty but due to the religious based practice. How to cope with these problems on the patients with rooted belief and behaviors based on religions is challenging. This main query needs systematic approach to find the solution.

The final case is a case detected in a rural village. Of interest, in this village, all except on child had malnutrition. This village is far from the city and very poor. So what contribute to the exceptional one case. The body is not malnutriented but very fat. The overweight is indicated. This boy is the son of the head of this village. His family is the richest family in the village and has enough money to pay for excessive foods for the family. This is the cause of excessive desert ingestion of the identified problematic case. Despite the high rate of malnutrition in this village, the case of overweight, the totally different problem can be seen. The totally discrepancy can be detected. Howe to cope with this fact is also the main query. In addition, this can bring us to the specific caution. It is required to look for both sides of a scenario because the coin has two faces. Coping with a case in the community needs gently thought and careful consideration.

Finally the author hereby would like to talk about the concept of holistic "bio-psycho-social [15 – 20]" approach. This is the new proved useful concept. The interrelationship between bio, psycho and social factors is approved. This means effects of social backgrounds on both biological and psychological appearances of everyone. For example, poverty can bring malnutrition due to the fact that there is no money to buy anything to eat. Poverty can also makes the affected subjects become anxious and developed symptoms due to stress. Therefore, the approach for any problem must base on the concept of bio-psyo-social approach.

Infection: What It Is?

Infection is a specific group of medical disorder. Infection means the condition that human body is infected by pathogenic organism. The pathogenic organism in this scenario can be fungus, virus, bacteria or parasite. However, sometimes we called the infection by parasite as infestation. Also, somebody do not accept that viral infection is an actual infection because virus is considered not a living organism and accepted as only a particle. Considering the pathophysiology process of infection, it must start from the triad of interrelationship: host, organism and environment. If there is no proper situation to allow the interrelationship, good conditions of the three factors, there will not be and must not be infection. Infectious organism must have enough virulence to cause infection. Host must be prone to the infection. Finally, the environment must be appropriate to allow contact between host and agent and both host and organism must live in the same environment, if not the infection will not occur.

Human host get pathogen from several external environments. The pathogen has to face up with the defensive mechanism of host. This can be primarily by non specific, non immune, system. The examples are mucous secretion and natural reflex such as cough for pushing away the pathogen out of the respirator tract. If the pathogen can pass the primary defense, it has to face up with another defensive mechanism, the immune system. The immune system has its specific characteristics. It has the memory and specificity. Both cellular and humoral immune response work altogether to help get rid of the pathogen. Concerning the act of cellular immunity, T cell plays its important role in the action. The main substance for this system is the cytokine. Concerning the act of humoral immunity, B cell plays its important role in the action. The main substance for the system is the antibody or immunoglobulin (either Ig G, Ig A, IgM or IgE). If the immune system fails to get rid of and control of alien organism, the pathogen can be successfully invade into the human host and cause the problem and it finally reach the stage of infection. The pathology is caused by the success in invasion of the problematic pathogenic organism. Looking at any infection, the basic clinical presentation is the inflammation [21 - 22]. This can be the cardinal sign of infection describing as pain, swelling, redness and hot. Additional signs and symptoms can be seen. The common presentations are due to the passing of content from body orifice which is corresponding to that infection. For example, sputum production can be seen in respiratory tract infection and watery stool passing can be seen in gastrointestinal tract infection.

At present, there are thousands of documented infectious diseases. There are many and many problems due to infection. It can be said that all countries around the world have the problem of infectious diseases. This implies the importance of infectious disease in present medicine. To mange infection is the concept. The two necessary tools for management are the investigation by laboratory tests or imaging technology and the treatment by either medicine, surgery or other means of treatment. Diagnosis can be done by good investigation and can be the tool to detect the cause of infection. The aim of diagnosis is mainly to identify the problematic pathogen. This can be the detection of the pathogen directly or can be the indirect determination of parts of pathogen (antigen) or human body response to the pathogen (antibody). The therapy is the tool to get rid of and control of pathogen. For treatment, it should be noted that some pathogens can be treated, however, the other are presently not. The treatment for the non treatable disease might be the direction for relieving of the symptoms that called symptomatic treatment. The examples of non treatable diseases are viral encephalitis disorders such as rabies.

In addition to the diagnosis and treatment, there is also another important medical facet to cope with the infection. The prevention must be mentioned. Indeed, many infectious diseases, nearly all, can be preventable before the exact episode of infection. The prevention can be primary, secondary or tertiary mode. However, the most important prevention for many infectious diseases is the vaccination, which is concerned as a primary prevention. Several vaccines are available at present and new vaccines are underdeveloped to counteract with the problematic infectious diseases [23 – 26].

Emerging of Infectious Disease [27 - 35]

The infectious disease is problematic in medicine. However, the cluster of infections that appears in one times seems to be more problematic. The outbreak or epidemic of infectious disease usually causes the cluster of patients loading to the local health care workers. It is the basic concept in preventive medicine to control and perform routine surveillance on important infectious disease. Deep investigation on each disease outbreak is recommended and can help analyze for the rooted cause for that specific outbreak. This process can lead to the planning for proper corrective and preventive act5ion. The area with the common appearance of an infectious disease is called as the endemic area for that infection. However, there is another fact to be concerned. This is emerging of infectious disease. Emerging seems the problematic condition that needs careful concern. In medicine, there are three conditions of emerging of infectious diseases. The first kind is new emerging infectious disease. This is the condition of new appearance of infectious diseases. The examples are H5N1 bird flu infection in human beings, SARS infection in human beings and Nipah virus infection in human beings. Please note that the author uses the phase "in human beings" in all mentioned new emerging infectious diseases. This is due to the fact that the described infectious diseases are not the new diseases but old infections in animal but firstly affect human beings. Indeed, the three mentioned diseases in this stage are believed to be due to the process of zoonosis. Zoonosis is usually the condition relating to new emerging infectious disease in human beings [36]. There are many factors contributing to this fact. These include environmental change due to global warming that permit the extension of spreading of the pathogenic organisms and the human behavior. Considering the human behavior, human beings are at risk because their bad practice. For example, invasion into the forest in Africa by human beings is believed to be the starting point for present HIV infection.

The second problematic condition of emerging of infectious disease is called remerging infectious disease. It should be noted that some infectious disease are already managed in medicine for a long time due to the medical control program. However, in some days, these diseases can be emerged again. This brings the term of remerging infectious disease. The best example is the condition of remerging tuberculosis in HIV infected case. The fact is that the immune is severely impaired in the affected HIV seropositive case. The CD4+ positive cells are destroyed and lead to the condition of immunodeficiency. This can make the infection of tuberculous agent to be easy.

The third final condition of emerging of infectious disease is called intended emerging infectious disease. Why it is intended? This can be easily explained in the condition of bioterrorism [37 – 38]. Due to the conflict in the present day, bioterrorism can be expected. Many infectious agents can be used as bioterrorism agents. The good examples are anthrax and arbovirus. The best well known condition of this kind of emerging of infectious disease is the report on the contamination of anthrax in the envelope of the letter that distributed widely in USA [39 - 40]. This can be the focus of medical interest in the present era of terrorism.

It is accepted that emerging of infectious disease is a famous concern in public health. As already mentioned, emerging infectious disease is usually undetectable at the first time and do not covered by the existed surveillance program. It cannot be exactly impress that what the actual pathogenic organism is at the first appearance. Every country must have its specific health care sector to cope with the infectious disease and possible emerging of infectious disease. The unit is usually called Center of Disease Control or CDC. When an emerging of infectious disease is noticed, CDC must play important role for management. CDC usually takes part in primary management of the episode. The method in preventive medicine can be and usually be applied. The aim of the response to emerging infectious disease is primarily to cope with the problem. Firstly, the control or limitation of the problem is the first attempt in the acute phase. The basic problem must be solved at first. Limitation of extension of disease must be at high attempt. The identification of the problem must be rapidly done to help limit the specific site of problematic attack of the disease. When the area is successfully closed, the next step is to find the pathogenic organism. This can be done by several laboratory investigation techniques. The focused disease surveillance must be done. If the pathogen is identified, quaranteen can be more effective. Rooted cause analysis to detect the exact pathogenic organism and pathogenesis process must be further done. If the nature of emerging infectious disease can be detected or discovered, it should be used immediately for planning for control although the exact pathogen is not already approved. This will effectively help control the condition. For example, at first, the H5N1 infection is not already known but it is clarified that this is a respiratory tract disease, therefore, the public health care sector launched the specific protocol to cope with the problem based on basic principle for control of respiratory infection for this new disease [41 – 42]. It should be noted that the collaboration between public health care sections is needed. Multidisciplinary approach can help reduce the problem. In addition, the international collaboration can also help learn the situation. Often, the new techniques from other countries can help identify the problem and lead to succeed in management. Routinely, the exact determination of actual pathogen takes time and its takes more time to find the proper treatment of the new disease. The control of spreading of disease seems to be more important. Basic infection control rules can be used as previously mentioned. In addition, the surveillance system must be set as further preventive action. With the already described process, the management of emerging of infectious disease can be successfully done.

In addition, when approach to an emerging of infectious disease, the concept of social geography should be used. This must cover all aspects of that disease. For example, if consider on a new emerging disease that is due to eating, the most interesting aspects of that disease, which relate to the technology, economics and regulation of the (mainly processed) food chain and to consumer behavior, are unlikely to be captured by a purely descriptive geographical approach.

Last but not least, it should be mentioned for the importance of health education. Basically, population will be at risk if they do not practice in the correct way [43]. The fact to be noted is that practice results from belief and belief results from knowledge. If there is no good knowledge, it cannot be expected for good practice. Therefore, the health education is needed to create the proper good health behavior of the population. Indeed, health education must be taught in the school and generalized to general population in the communities. In the case of emerging of infectious disease, the basic concept of infection control has to be taught to the general population. This is the least required health knowledge for them. When there are more clear evidences on the disease, more information should be and must be given to them as additional session. The media must be wide and easily assessed such as TV. The knowledge must be easy as what to do and what not to do in the situation of emerging of infectious disease. This can help relief the panic of the population to the emerging of infectious disease [44].

Conclusion

India or South Asia is accepted as a pearl area in medicine. BMJ recently publish a special issue on medicine in this area. The proposed book focuses on the "Emerging and remerging infections in India", a new health problem, in the aspects relating to the tropical medicine. The book will cover specifically the clinical aspect, scientific laboratory aspect, public health aspect as well as the social sciences relating to emerging and remerging infections in East Asia context. Mainly the book will present summative data from the molecular to the population scales, as well as additional metanalysis for important topics. In addition, the diagnostic guideline and clinical practice guideline of the mentioned conditions will be presented. The academic level of this book is aimed to be for the wide range from the medical student, resident, general practitioner, specialist in infectious and tropical medicine and the researchers in medical sciences. It can also be useful for the medical personnel in allied health sciences. Due to the globalization in the present day, the change in the epidemiology of diseases from one site to the others all around the world can be expected. Indian story is the focus of interest in medicine. The summative on the common infectious problems in the tropical countries can be and should be performed. This work can be a useful reference material for the practitioners who are not familiar to the unique problems of the developing world and might face up with those problems due to the possible migration of diseases. The proposed book can make them at least realize and familial with the problems.

References

[1] Tharyan P, Ghersi D. Registering clinical trials in India: a scientific and ethical imperative. *Natl Med J India*. 2008 Jan-Feb;21(1):31-4.

[2] Trunkey DD. The medical world is flat too. World J Surg. 2008 Aug;32(8):1583-604.

[3] Bhargava A, Chatterjee B. Chikungunya fever, falciparum malaria, dengue fever, Japanese encephalitis... are we listening to the warning signs for public health in India? *Indian J Med Ethics*. 2007 Jan-Mar;4(1):18-23.

[4] Saiyed HN, Tiwari RR. Occupational health research in India. Ind *Health*. 2004 Apr;42(2):141-8.

[5] John TJ. Emerging & re-emerging bacterial pathogens in India. *Indian J Med Res*. 1996 Jan;103:4-18.

[6] Antia NH. On health and healing: community health care in India. *Indian J Pediatr*. 1991 Mar-Apr;58(2):161-73.

[7] Wiwanitkit V. Secondary and tertiary structure aberration of alpha globin chain in haemoglobin Q-India disorder. *Indian J Pathol Microbiol*. 2006 Oct;49(4):491-4.

[8] Muniyandi M, Ramachandran R. Socioeconomic inequalities of tuberculosis in India. *Expert Opin Pharmacother*. 2008 Jul;9(10):1623-8.

[9] Ramaraj R, Alpert JS._Indian poverty and cardiovascular disease. *Am J Cardiol*. 2008 Jul 1;102(1):102-6.

[10] Dror DM, van Putten-Rademaker O, Koren R. Cost of illness: evidence from a study in five resource-poor locations in India. *Indian J Med Res*. 2008 Apr;127(4):347-61.

[11] Kumar D, Goel NK, Kalia M, Swami HM, Singh R. Gap between awareness and practices regarding maternal and child health among women in an urban slum community. *Indian J Pediatr*. 2008 May;75(5):455-8.

[12] Bose K, Bisai S, Chakraborty J, Datta N, Banerjee P. Extreme levels of underweight and stunting among pre-adolescent children of low socioeconomic class from Madhyamgram and Barasat, West Bengal, India. *Coll Antropol*. 2008 Mar;32(1):73-7.

[13] McDermott E, Selman L, Wright M, Clark D. Hospice and palliative care development in India: a multimethod review of services and experiences. *J Pain Symptom Manage*. 2008 Jun;35(6):583-93.

[14] Srivastava NM, Awasthi S, Mishra R. Neonatal morbidity and care-seeking behavior in urban Lucknow. *Indian Pediatr*. 2008 Mar;45(3):229-32.

[15] Sabbioni ME. Is a bio-psycho-social approach in cancer research feasible? *Ann Oncol*. 1993 Nov;4(9):714-5

[16] Rickelman B. Bio-psycho-social linguistics: a conceptual approach to nurse-patient interaction. *Nurs Res*. 1971 Sep-Oct;20(5):398-403.

[17] Branzei PP, Nathanson IN. The bio-psycho-social tridimensional constructivism of Socolas' School in the perspective of contemporary psychiatry (author's transl). *Acta Psychiatr Belg*. 1981 Sep-Oct;81(5):425-36.

[18] La Malfa G, Campigli M, Bertelli M, Mangiapane A, Cabras PL. The psychopathological model of mental retardation: theoretical and therapeutic considerations. *Res Dev Disabil*. 1997 Nov-Dec;18(6):407-13.

[19] Zikmund V. Problems with the limitations of medicine. *Bratisl Lek Listy*. 1995 Feb;96(2):63-8.

[20] Worrall L. Professionalism and functional outcomes. *J Commun Disord*. 2006 Jul-Aug;39(4):320-7.

[21] Medzhitov R. Origin and physiological roles of inflammation. *Nature*. 2008 Jul 24;454(7203):428-35.

[22] Libby P. Inflammatory mechanisms: the molecular basis of inflammation and disease. *Nutr Rev*. 2007 Dec;65(12 Pt 2):S140-6.

[23] Stinchfield PK. Practice-proven interventions to increase vaccination rates and broaden the immunization season. *Am J Med*. 2008 Jul;121(7 Suppl 2):S11-21.

[24] Ackerman LK. Update on immunizations in children and adolescents. *Am Fam Physician*. 2008 Jun 1;77(11):1561-8.

[25] Expanded programme on immunization (EPI) immunization schedules in the WHO Western Pacific Region, 1995. *Wkly Epidemiol Rec*. 1996 May 3;71(18):133-7.

[26] Middleton DB, Zimmerman RK, Mitchell KB. Vaccine schedules and procedures, 2007. *J Fam Pract*. 2007 Feb;56(2 Suppl Vaccines):S47-60, C4-8.

[27] Pekosz A, Glass GE. Emerging viral diseases. *Md Med*. 2008 Winter;9(1):11, 13-6.

[28] Okamoto Y, Nagai Y. The program of Founding Research Centers for Emerging and Reemerging Infectious Diseases: the present status and future prospects. *Uirusu*. 2007 Dec;57(2):207-15.

[29] Mizutani T. Establishment of a system for determination of emerging infectious diseases (RDV method), and its application. *Uirusu*. 2007 Dec;57(2):217-25.

[30] Nicolasora N, Kaul DR. Infectious disease emergencies. *Med Clin North Am*. 2008 Mar;92(2):427-41, x

[31] Rodier G, Greenspan AL, Hughes JM, Heymann DL. Global public health security. *Emerg Infect Dis*. 2007 Oct;13(10):1447-52.

[32] Peetermans WE, De Munter P. Emerging and re-emerging infectious diseases. *Acta Clin Belg*. 2007 Sep-Oct;62(5):337-41.

[33] Taniguchi K. Emerging and re-emerging infectious diseases. *Nippon Rinsho*. 2005 Apr;63 Suppl 4:540-5.

[34] Global surveillance of emerging and re-emerging diseases. *Wkly Epidemiol Rec*. 2001 Jul 20;76(29):218-24.

[35] Infectious diseases. Some recent threats. *Health Care Food Nutr Focus*. 2006 Jan;23(1):9-12.

[36] Antonijević B, Madle-Samardzija N, Turkulov V, Canak G, Gavrancić C, Petrović-Milosević I. Zoonoses--a current issue in contemporary infectology. *Med Pregl*. 2007 Sep-Oct;60(9-10):441-3.

[37] Nordin JD, Kasimow S, Levitt MJ, Goodman MJ._Bioterrorism surveillance and privacy: intersection of HIPAA, the Common Rule, and public health law. *Am J Public Health*. 2008 May;98(5):802-7

[38] Richard JL, Grimes DE._Bioterrorism: class A agents and their potential presentations in immunocompromised patients. *Clin J Oncol Nurs*. 2008 Apr;12(2):295-302.

[39] Shadomy SV, Smith TL. Zoonosis update. Anthrax. *J Am Vet Med Assoc*. 2008 Jul 1;233(1):63-72.

[40] Dance A. FBI to reveal anthrax data. *Nature*. 2008 Aug 21;454(7207):928.

[41] Dash S, Albrecht H._Management of avian influenza H5N1--diagnosis, treatment, and vaccination. *J S C Med Assoc*. 2008 Jun;104(5):141-5

[42] Thanh TT, Doorn HR, de Jong MD._Human H5N1 influenza: Current insight into pathogenesis. *Int J Biochem Cell Biol*. 2008;40(12):2671-4.

[43] Allen PJ._The world awaits the next pandemic: will it be H5N1, the 'bird flu'? *J Child Health Care*. 2006 Sep;10(3):178-87.

[44] Hayes P. When fear becomes panic. *Clin Nurs Res*. 2003 Nov;12(4):299-303.

Chapter II

Leptospirosis in India

Introduction to Leptospirosis [1 - 22]

Leptospirosis is an important spirochete infection. The pathogenic organism is a spiral or helical shaped prokaryote and is an obligate aerobe that is highly motile. Concerning the natural history of this infection, the pathogenic organism which is excreted in urine by rats and other infected mammals can be transmitted in contaminated water, usually flood water. The infected person gets the germ by direct contact with a skin wound, especially at the foot. Not wearing shoes and walking in flood water is a risk-filled behavior for this infection. Leptospirosis is an important tropical disease with high prevalence in many tropical countries [1]. Presenting symptoms vary with age: children showing primarily fever, vomiting, headache, abdominal and generalized muscle pain and diarrhea while adults usually have fever, headache, anorexia, myalgia and constipation [2 - 3]. However, fever is the main symptom and can be misdiagnosed with other common tropical infections which usually present with fever. Myalgia, especially at the calf, is also common. Also, this can be mimicked by other common tropical infections.

Renal involvement is a common complication of leptospirosis. Bacterial invasion, inflammatory process, hemodynamic alterations and direct toxicity of bacterial products are thought to be responsible for the development of nephropathy [4]. The pathogenesis of renal pathology in leptospirosis is not well clarified and is still the topic for further research in tropical nephrology. Pathologically, all renal structures are involved. Interstitial nephritis is the basic lesion, and is observed even in patients without clinical renal manifestations and tubular necrosis is the important pathological counterpart of acute renal failure [4]. For the case with renal failure, standard management as that for other causes of renal failure is required. The usages of dialysis for management of such cases are recommended. Chronic renal failure is not common in this disease.

In addition, jaundice is another important finding of leptospirosis. Hepatitis due to leptospirosis is a concern, and leptospirosis should be a differential diagnosis in tropical jaundice. For the leptospirosis hepatitis, jaundice is the common clinical manifestation. The histopathology of the leptospirosis hepatitis is similar to those seen in the cholestatic type of viral hepatitis; however, the histopathologic changes are not seriously impaired. Most of the biopsied specimens during the first week usually have general minimal changes and the histopathological changes of the liver are more pronounced, including eosinophilic necrosis and mononuclear cell infiltration, in the next week. During the fourth and the fifth week, the changes are very slight. However, luckily, most patients present a mild clinical form of leptospirosis, which consists of a self-limited febrile process, without jaundice. Nevertheless, about one fifth of patients suffer severe infections, with intense jaundice [16]. For prevention, because of its dependence on animal carrier contact, leptospirosis is accepted to be a disease of poverty. Underprivileged people in the rural endemic area are at risk of being infected with leptospirosis. Also, it causes economical loss and impacts social functions. The monitoring of the incidence of the disease provides useful data for disease surveillancc and control.

Nephrogenic Property of Pathogenic Leptospira, Does it Exist or Not?

Introduction

Yang et al showed that outer membrane proteins (OMPs) of pathogenic leptospira activated nuclear NFkappaB binding and stimulated downstream inducible nitric oxide (iNOS), monocyte chemoattractant protein-1 (MCP-1) and tumor necrosis factor-alpha (TNF-alpha) expression [23]. They indicated that leptospiral infection might induce tubulo-interstitial nephritis through a toxic component in the outer membrane followed by expression of inflammatory genes [23]. However, the underlying pathophysiology of nephritis as well as renal failure in leptospirosis is not well documented. Here, the author used a genomic technology to investigate the nephritogenic property of pathogenic leptospira.

Materials and Methods

The author uses the bioinformatic technique in order to investigate the homologue of the reference nephritogenic protein sequence to pathologic leptospira genome. A blast search using the NCBI blast tool (http://www.ncbi.nlm.nih.gov/blast/) was performed. The standard nephritogenic protein sequence is NM_198640 or *Mus musculus* expressed sequence AI324046 (nephritogenic protein). The genome of *Leptospira interrogans* serovar Lai str. (56601) was used as a blasted genome.

Results

The homology investigation between NM_198640 (1684 letters) and 56601 (4,691,184 total letters) was performed. Gap Penalties parameters are: Existence = 0 and Extension = 0. According to this study, no significant similarity was found.

Discussion

Leptospirosis is a spirochaetal zoonotic disease. It is a worldwide zoonosis caused by pathogenic Leptospira species, for which humans are accidental hosts. It is endemic in the tropical urban areas including our country, where seasonal epidemics are becoming increasingly common [3]. Laboratory tests are necessary to confirm the diagnosis of clinically suspected leptospirosis owing to its varied symptomatology [3].Considering leptospirosis nephropathy, the clinical spectrum of renal manifestations include mild urinary sediment change, hypokalemia, tubular dysfunction, decreased response to fluid load and acute renal failure (ARF) [4]. ARF reflects the severity of leptospirosis, is catabolic, and is commonly associated with cholestatic jaundice [4]. Visith and Kearkiat noted that severe renal failure may be complicated by multiple organ involvement [4].

Microbiologically, some bacteria contain nephritogenic protein and this protein can lead to the pathology of kidney. A good example is *Streptococcus* spp [24]. In renal failure, due to nephritogenic protein of *Streptoccus* spp, the diagnosis is usually not difficult when a nephritic clinical presentation (along with such manifestations as hematuria, edema, and hypertension) is associated with serologic evidence of recent streptococcal infection and a depressed serum complement concentration. In leptospirosis, the nephritis can be seen. Recently, Yener and Keles said that the detected incidence of infection with *L. interrogans* was not high, but there was a relationship between the presence of interstitial nephritis and leptospiral antigens [25]. Sitprija et al said that bacterial invasion and toxicity of the outer membrane with generation of cytokines, chemokines, and cellular infiltration were important in cellular injury [26]. However, the evidence of nephrogenic property of pathogenic leptospira has never been verified.

Here, the author studied whether the nephritogenic property exists in pathogenic leptospira, *Leptospira interrogans*. The author uses a bioinformatic method to identify the homology within the genome of pathologic leptospira to the standard reference nephritogenic protein. Of interest, no homology can be seen. Hence, it might conclude that there is no nephritogenic property for the studied pathologic leptospira. The nephritis in the leptospira renal failure might be due the other pathological process, and not directly linked to the leptospira sequence, such as in hemodynamic alteration. Further studies on the pathogenesis of nephritis and renal failure in leptospirosis infection are warranted.

The Leptospira Organism and Leptospiral Immune Complex, are these Responsible for Renal Pathology?

Introduction

Renal involvement is a common complication of leptospirosis. Bacterial invasion, inflammatory process, hemodynamic alterations and direct toxicity of bacterial products are thought to be responsible for the development of nephropathy [21]. Histologically, all renal structures are involved. Interstitial nephritis is a basic lesion, and is observed even in patients without clinical manifestations [21]. Yener and Keles said that the incidence of leptospirosis was not high, but there was a relationship between presence of interstitial nephritis and leptospiral antigens [27]. However, exact underlying pathophysiology of nephritis in leptospirosis is not well described. Recently, Galli et al proposed that the presence of high concentrations of circulating immune complexes only during the acute phase of illness seems to confirm that in leptospirosis, immune complex reactions are a significant pathogenetic element [28]. In addition, van den et al proposed an immune-mediated process with immune complex formation and binding and activation of complements resulting in leukocytosis, thrombotic glomerulopathy, endothelial alteration and haemorrhagcs [29]. However, the exact correlation between the leptospiral immune complex and renal pathology has never been clarified.

Materials and Methods

Here, the author reviewed the reported size of the renal arteriole, glomerular pore size, the molecular size of leptospira organism and immunoglobulin in the literature. The basic concept that larger objects cannot pass through the smaller diameter vessels is applied.

Results

The molecular sizes of the leptospira organism and leptospiral-Ig complex are 300 nm and about 305 nm (10 nm of streptococcus group A [30] and 5 nm of immunoglobulin [30]), respectively. The diameters of renal afferent and efferent arterioles are about 200 nm. The glomerular pore size is 4.0 - 4.5 nm [30]. The size of the leptospira organism and leptospiral-Ig complex is larger than both renal arterioles and glomerular pore size.

Discussion

Leptospirosis is a re-emerging infectious disease that occurs in the canine population in urban and rural environments. It is caused by a filamentous spiral bacterium that has a predilection for renal tubules partially resulting in nephropathology. Acute renal failure, hepatic dysfunction, and hemorrhagic diathesis are the most common clinical signs of leptospirosis [1 - 20]. Although the nephropathology is a hallmark of leptospirosis, there has been no clarification on the exact pathogenesis. Since immune complex is a possible pathogenic mechanism in leptospirosis, it might be a corresponding underlying cause for renal disorder in leptospirosis. Here, the author investigates the feasibility of leptospiral immune complex as the underlying cause of leptospiral nephropathy.

Here, the author uses a basic consideration in nanostructure of the kidney and organism for further implication. Of interest, the size of the leptospira organism and leptospiral-Ig complex is larger than both renal arterioles and glomerular pore size. This can imply that either the organism or leptospiral-Ig complex can pass into the renal arteriole. Although the size of immune complex is larger than the glomerular pore size, which implies the possibility of rodding and cause of further immunopathology, the immune complex size is larger than the renal arteriole, hence it cannot enter into the glomerulus to cause the rodding. The findings in this work can support the fact that there has been no report on the identification of the organism or immune complex in leptospiral nephropathy. The author proposed that the possible exact mechanism of leptospiral nephropathy might be a toxin. Indeed, Sitprija et al said that bacterial invasion and toxicity of the outer membrane with generation of cytokines, chemokines, and cellular infiltration were important cellular injuries [26]. In addition, Yang et al found that outer membrane proteins of pathogenic leptospira activated nuclear NFkappaB binding and stimulated downstream inducible nitric oxide, monocyte chemoattractant protein-1 and tumor necrosis factor-alpha expression [23]. They indicated that the infection might induce tubulo-interstitial nephritis through a toxic component in the outer membrane followed by expression of inflammatory genes [23].

Leptospirosis in India

Leptospirosis infection is an important vector-borne disease. With an annual incidence of millions of clinically diagnosed cases, leptospirosis infection is still one of the main spirochete infections in the world. This reflects a need for intensive pathogen control because leptospiros continues to affect a lot of global populations in the tropical regions of the world. Asia is an area dealing with this infection. The endemic areas of leptospirosis cover some specific areas in the Asian region. South Asia is an area confirming the problem of leptospirosis. In this chapter, the author uses the specific term of Indian leptospirosis to describe the problem of leptospirosisin in South Asia.

1. Leptospirosis in India

India is a big country. There are also some areas that lie in the tropical region. Therefore, the problem of leptospirosis can be seen. The leptospirosis can be classified as an important emerging infection in India. There are many reports on emerging of leptospirosis in India as shown in Table 1.

2. Leptospirosis in Nepal

Nepal is another country in South Asia. There are no reports on the emergence of leptospirosis in Nepal. This might be due to the fact that Nepal is not in the tropical area of Asia.

Table 1. Reports on the emergence of leptospirosis in India.

Author	Details
Masali et al [31]	*Masali et al reported on* control and prevention of Leptospirosis outbreak in six villages of Raichur district, Karnataka, India [31].
Vijayachari et al [32]	*Vijayachari* et al reported on leptospirosis in the Andaman Islands, India [32].
De et al [33]	De et al reported on an outbreak of leptospirosis in Mumbai, India [33].
Chandrasekaran [34]	*Chandrasekaran* reported on an outbreak of leptospirosis in Mumbai, India [34]
Maskey et al [35]	*Maskey* et al reported on leptospirosis in Mumbai focusing on post-deluge outbreak 2005 scenario [35].
Karande et al [36]	*Karande* et al reported on concurrent outbreak of leptospirosis and dengue in Mumbai, India, 2002 [36].
Vijayachari et al [37]	*Vijayachari* et al reported on leptospirosis among schoolchildren of the Andaman and Nicobar Islands, India and mentioned low levels of morbidity and mortality among pre-exposed children during an epidemic [37].
Jena et al [38]	*Jena* et al reported on an outbreak of leptospirosis in Orissa, India: the importance of surveillance [38].
Pappachan et al [39]	*Pappachan* et al reported on relation of rainfall pattern and epidemic leptospirosis in the Indian state of Kerala [39].
Ramakrishnan et al [40]	*Ramakrishnan et al reported on* an institutional outbreak of leptospirosis in Chennai, South India [40].
Bharadwaj et al [41]	*Bharadwaj* et al reported on an urban outbreak of leptospirosis in Mumbai, India [41].
Joshi et al [42]	*Joshi* et al reported on the role of IgM specific indirect immunofluorescence assay in diagnosing an outbreak of leptospirosis [42].
Karande et al [43]	*Karande* et al reported on leptospirosis in children in Mumbai slums [43].
Sehgal et al [44]	*Sehgal* et al reported on an outbreak of leptospirosis after the cyclone in Orissa [44].
CDC [45]	Report of the investigation of a post-cyclone outbreak in Orissa, November 1999 was published [45].
Venkataraman and Nedunchelliyan [46]	*Venkataraman and Nedunchelliyan*_reported on epidemiology of an outbreak of leptospirosis in man and dog [46].
Srivastava [47]	*Srivastava* reported on outbreak of Weil's disease in a food fad commune in India [47].
Singh [48]	*Singh* reported on outbreak of Weil's disease in a food fad commune in India [48].
*Agrawal and Srivastava*_[49]	*Agrawal and Srivastava*_reported on an outbreak of Weil's disease in a food fad commune in India [49]..
Ratnam et al [50]	*Ratnam et al reported on*_serological evidence of leptospirosis in a human population following an outbreak of the disease in cattle [50].
Mukherjea et al [51]	*Mukherjea* et al reported on an outbreak of leptospirosis in Howrah, West Bengal [51].

3. Leptospirosis in Bhutan

Bhutan is another country in South Asia. There is no report on the emergence of leptospirosis in Bhutan. This might be due to the fact that Bhutan is not in the tropical area of Asia.

4. Leptospirosis in Maldives

Maldives is another country in South Asia. Of interest, there are no reports on emerging of leptospirosis in Maldives although this country lies in the tropical zone. This might be due to the fact that this country is a combination of several islands in the Indian Ocean.

5. Leptospirosis in Sri Lanka

Sri Lanka is another country in South Asia. There is no report on the emergence of leptospirosis in Sri Lanka.

6. Leptospirosis in Bangladesh

Bangladesh is another country in South Asia. There is no report on the emergence of leptospirosis in Bangladesh.

7. Leptospirosis in Pakistan

Pakistan is another country in South Asia. However, there is no report on the emergence of leptospirosis in Pakistan. This may be due to the fact that this area is far from the monsoon.

In summary, the common appearance of outbreaks is rainy season. Flooding is the main risk situation. Indeed, the climate as monsoon type in tropical Asia can bring several storm every year and this can lead to flood. When wandering rats are limited in a locked place due to flooding, it can pass the infected urine into the water and can be the source of infection. This can be the problem to the local people who live in the flood area. There is a fact that rat and the poverty usually live in the same place. The poverty is at higher risk than the rich. They have to live and walk in the contaminated water and can get infection. The other fact to be mentioned is the occupation of the local occupation of the people in tropical Asia. Agriculture is the main occupation. The work in the paddy field can be a risk behavior. Because, the farmers usually wear no shoes when working in the water in their paddy fields, this can bring the risk for infection if there is contamination in the water in those fields. Providing specific health education to the risk population is required. Promotion of wearing shoes is the focus. This might be the clue for succeed in management of leptospirosis in this area. Finally, global warming which is the present world problem can also bring high risk for emerging of leptospirosis because this can bring more frequent attack of monsoon. This is the topic in present medicine.

Blood Exchange, a Useful Treatment for Acute Renal Failure in Weil's Disease [52 – 58]

Weil's is the most serious form of leptospiral infection. High death rate from this condition is reported in medical literature. It has high fatality and morbidity and even the supportive and symptomatic treatments cannot reduce the severity of the disease [26]. Severe hyperbilirubinemia induced acute renal failure is the hallmark of this specific disease. The role of blood exchange in the therapy of leptospirosis has not been defined, although it has anecdotally been used in subjects with favorable clinical outcomes [52 – 57]. Here, the author performs this mini-research in order to summarize the outcomes of blood exchange among reported Thai acute renal failure cases owing to Weil's disease. A literature review on the papers concerning blood exchange among Thai acute renal failure patients owing to Weil's disease was performed from the database of the published works cited in the Index Medicus and Science Citation Index and also the published works in all 256 local Thai journals, which are not covered by the international citation index. The reports that had no complete data were excluded for further analysis.

According to this review, there were 5 reports [53 - 57] containing data of 17 Thai ARF patients (average age = 38.5 $\pm$ 7.9 years) owing to Weil's disease. The average duration of illness of the patients is 8.3 $\pm$ 3.2 days. The average pre-exchange BUN, creatinine (Cr), total bilirubin (TB) and direct bilirubin (DB) levels are 68.7 $\pm$ 33.5 mg/dL, 5.0 $\pm$ 2.0 mg/dL, 29.7 $\pm$ 7.0 mg/dL and 16.3 $\pm$ 7.5 mg/dL orderly. All patients also received standard antibiotic therapy accompanied with blood exchange. The average blood usage is 7900.0 $\pm$ 1354.4 mL. The average pre-exchange BUN, Creatinine, total bilirubin and direct bilirubin levels were equal to 68.7 $\pm$ 33.5 mg/dL, 5.0 $\pm$ 2.0 mg/dL, 29.7 $\pm$ 7.0 mg/dL and 16.3 $\pm$ 7.5 mg/dL respectively. The average pre-exchange BUN, Cr, TB and DB levels were equal to 59.6 $\pm$ 11.7 mg/dL, 4.6 $\pm$ 2.2 mg/dL, 15.1 $\pm$ 4.1 mg/dL and 7.5 $\pm$ 2.4 mg/dL orderly. A statistical significant reduction of TB and DB but not for BUN and Cr can be seen. Of the 17 patients, all had complete and full recovery. These observations suggest that blood exchange is helpful in treating acute renal failure associated with Weil's disease. The reduction of bilirubin is the corresponding therapeutic mechanism of blood exchange. Blood exchange, in addition to conventional treatment, is accepted as helpful management in severe leptospirosis with complications and hyperbilirubinemia.

Correlation between Rainfall and Prevalence of Leptospirosis [59 - 62]

The human infection with leptospira spirochete is common in many tropical countries. The surveys of the disease's prevalence are helpful for prevention and control of disease and have been continuously performed in endemic areas. The correlation between rainfall and prevalence of leptospirosis has been proposed by Pappachan et al [61]. Kupek et al also noted that rainfall, a sensitive indicator of large amounts of rain falling in a brief period of time, is a useful predictor for the prevalence of leptospirosis [63]. Indeed, large outbreaks of leptospirosis have occurred following excess rainfall, and the following exposure to fresh water during occupational agricultural activities [59 - 62]. Of interest, there was a recent report on the seasonal variation on the leptospirosis prevalence in Thailand, which indicated the peak prevalence occurring in the rainy season when the rainfall is very high [64]. In conclusion, the prevalence of leptospirosis infection in Thailand may depend on rainfall. Therefore, the surveillance and control of mosquitos during the period with high rainfall is recommended. However, it should be taken into account some other confounding factors, which also determine the transmission of leptospirosis, including other seasonal factors, like ambient temperature and humidity, before concluding that the increased prevalence is a result of rainfall alone. Further similar studies to assess the correlation between the rainfall and prevalence of infection in the other countries is required to fulfill the conclusion. In addition, the questions are more on the quantification of that effect and on the relationship with the emergence of outbreaks and on the impact of climate changes.

References

[1] Dutta TK, Christopher M. Leptospirosis--an overview. *J Assoc Physicians India.* 2005;53:545-51.

[2] Heisey GB, Nimmanitya S, Karnchanachetanee C, *et al.* Epidemiology and characterization of leptospirosis at an urban and provincial site in Thailand. Southeast Asian *J Trop Med Public Health.* 1988;19:317-22.

[3] *Sana AN, Shah S, Ahmad FM.* Laboratory diagnosis of leptospirosis. *J Postgrad Med* 2005;51:195-200.

[4] *Visith S, Kearkiat P.* Nephropathy in leptospirosis. *J Postgrad Med* 2005;51:184-8.

[5] *Yang CW, Wu MS, Pan MJ.* Leptospirosis renal disease. *Nephrol Dial Transplant.* 2001;16 Suppl 5:73-7.

[6] *Nissenson AR, Baraff LJ, Fine RN, Knutson DW.* Poststreptococcal acute glomerulonephritis: fact and controversy. *Ann Intern Med* 1979;91:76-86.

[7] *Yener Z, Keles H.* Immunoperoxidase and histopathological examinations of leptospiral nephritis in cattle. *J Vet Med A Physiol Pathol Clin Med.* 2001;48:441-7.

[8] *Sitprija V, Losuwanrak K, Kanjanabuch T.* Leptospiral nephropathy. *Semin Nephrol.* 2003;23:42-8.

[9] *Sumathi G, Narayanan R, Shivakumar S.* Leptospirosis laboratory, Madras Medical College: review of our experience (2004-2006). *Indian J Med Microbiol.* 2008 Apr-Jun;26(2):206-7

[10] *Yang CW.* Leptospirosis in Taiwan--an underestimated infectious disease. *Chang Gung Med J.* 2007 Mar-Apr;30(2):109-15.

[11] *Zunino M E, Pizarro P R.* Leptospirosis: a literature review. *Rev Chilena Infectol.* 2007 Jun;24(3):220-6.

[12] *Koizumi N, Watanabe H.* Leptospirosis. Nippon Rinsho. 2007 Mar 28;65 Suppl 3:200-3.

[13] *Palaniappan RU, Ramanujam S, Chang YF.* Leptospirosis: pathogenesis, immunity, and diagnosis. *Curr Opin Infect Dis*. 2007 Jun;20(3):284-92.

[14] *Vijayachari P, Sehgal SC.* Recent advances in the laboratory diagnosis of leptospirosis and characterisation of leptospires. *Indian J Med Microbiol*. 2006 Oct;24(4):320-2.

[15] *Sehgal SC.* Epidemiological patterns of leptospirosis. *Indian J Med Microbiol.* 2006 Oct;24(4):310-1.

[16] *Roca B.* Leptospirosis. *Rev Med Univ Navarra*. 2006 Apr-Jun;50(2):3-6.

[17] *Vickery B, Flynn SA, Calder L, Freebairn RC.* Leptospirosis presenting to an intensive care unit in provincial New Zealand: a case series and review. *Crit Care Resusc*. 2006 Sep;8(3):192-9.

[18] *John TJ.* The prevention and control of human leptospirosis. *J Postgrad Med.* 2005 Jul-Sep;51(3):205-9.

[19] *Kobayashi Y.* Human leptospirosis: management and prognosis. *J Postgrad Med.* 2005 Jul-Sep;51(3):201-4.

[20] *Ahmad SN, Shah S, Ahmad FM.* Laboratory diagnosis of leptospirosis. *J Postgrad Med*. 2005 Jul-Sep;51(3):195-200.

[21] *Visith S, Kearkiat P.* Nephropathy in leptospirosis. *J Postgrad Med.* 2005 Jul-Sep;51(3):184-8.

[22] Bal AM. Unusual clinical manifestations of leptospirosis. J Postgrad Med. 2005 Jul-Sep;51(3):179-83*Cachay ER, Vinetz JM.* A global research agenda for leptospirosis. J Postgrad Med. 2005 Jul-Sep;51(3):174-8.

[23] *Yang CW, Wu MS, Pan MJ.* Leptospirosis renal disease. *Nephrol Dial Transplant.* 2001;16 Suppl 5:73-7.

[24] *Nissenson AR, Baraff LJ, Fine RN, Knutson DW.* Poststreptococcal acute glomerulonephritis: fact and controversy. *Ann Intern Med* 1979;91:76-86.

[25] *Yener Z, Keles H.* Immunoperoxidase and histopathological examinations of leptospiral nephritis in cattle. *J Vet Med A Physiol Pathol Clin Med*. 2001;48:441-7.

[26] *Sitprija V, Losuwanrak K, Kanjanabuch T.* Leptospiral nephropathy. *Semin Nephrol.* 2003;23:42-8.

[27] Yener Z, Keles H. Immunoperoxidase and histopathological examinations of leptospiral nephritis in cattle. *J Vet Med A Physiol Pathol Clin Med* 2001;48:441-7

[28] Galli M, Esposito R, Crocchiolo P, Chemotti M, Gasparro M, Dall'Aglio Immune Complexes in Leptospirosis. *Infection.* 1985;13:156.

[29] van den Ingh TS, Hartman EG.}}}\f0\fs24 Pathology of acute Leptospira interrogans serotype icterohaemorrhagiae infection in the Syrian hamster. *Vet Microbiol.* 1986;12:367-76.

[30] Diem K, Lentner C. Scientific Table. 7 ed. *CIBAGEIGY:* Basle, 1971

[31] *Masali KA, Pulare MV, Kachare VK, Patil MB, Reddi S.* Control and prevention of rat fever (Leptospirosis) outbreak in six villages of Raichur district, Karnataka. *J Indian Med Assoc*. 2007 Nov;105(11):632, 634-6.

[32] *Vijayachari P, Sugunan AP, Sharma S, Roy S, Natarajaseenivasan K, Sehgal SC.* Leptospirosis in the Andaman Islands, India. *Trans R Soc Trop Med Hyg.* 2008 Feb;102(2):117-22

[33] De A, Varaiya A, Mathur M, Bhat M, Karande S, Yeolekar ME. An outbreak of leptospirosis in Mumbai. *Indian J Med Microbiol.* 2002 Jul-Sep;20(3):153-5.

[34] *Chandrasekaran S.* An outbreak of leptospirosis in Mumbai. *Indian J Med Microbiol.* 2003 Jan-Mar;21(1):63.

[35] *Maskey M, Shastri JS, Saraswathi K, Surpam R, Vaidya N.* Leptospirosis in Mumbai: post-deluge outbreak 2005. *Indian J Med Microbiol.* 2006 Oct;24(4):337-8

[36] *Karande S, Gandhi D, Kulkarni M, Bharadwaj R, Pol S, Thakare J, De A.* Concurrent outbreak of leptospirosis and dengue in Mumbai, India, 2002. *J Trop Pediatr.* 2005 Jun;51(3):174-81.

[37] *Vijayachari P, Sugunan AP, Murhekar MV, Sharma S, Sehgal SC.* Leptospirosis among schoolchildren of the Andaman & Nicobar Islands, India: low levels of morbidity and mortality among pre-exposed children during an epidemic. *Epidemiol Infect.* 2004 Dec;132(6):1115-20.

[38] *Jena AB, Mohanty KC, Devadasan N.* An outbreak of leptospirosis in Orissa, India: the importance of surveillance. *Trop Med Int Health.* 2004 Sep;9(9):1016-21.

[39] *Pappachan MJ, Sheela M, Aravindan KP.* Relation of rainfall pattern and epidemic leptospirosis in the Indian state of Kerala. *J Epidemiol Community Health.* 2004 Dec;58(12):1054.

[40] *Ramakrishnan R, Patel MS, Gupte MD, Manickam P, Venkataraghavan S.* An institutional outbreak of leptospirosis in Chennai, South India. *J Commun Dis.* 2003 Mar;35(1):1-8.

[41] *Bharadwaj R, Bal AM, Joshi SA, Kagal A, Pol SS, Garad G, Arjunwadkar V, Katti R.* An urban outbreak of leptospirosis in Mumbai, India. Jpn *J Infect Dis.* 2002 Dec;55(6):194-6.

[42] *Joshi S, Bal A, Bharadwaj R, Kumbhar R, Kagal A, Arjunwadkar V.* Role of IgM specific indirect immunofluorescence assay in diagnosing an outbreak of leptospirosis. *Indian J Pathol Microbiol.* 2002 Jan;45(1):75-7.

[43] *Karande S, Kulkarni H, Kulkarni M, De A, Varaiya A.* Leptospirosis in children in Mumbai slums. *Indian J Pediatr.* 2002 Oct;69(10):855-8.

[44] *Sehgal SC, Sugunan AP, Vijayachari P.* Outbreak of leptospirosis after the cyclone in Orissa. *Natl Med J India.* 2002 Jan-Feb;15(1):22-3.

[45] Leptospirosis, India. Report of the investigation of a post-cyclone outbreak in Orissa, November 1999. *Wkly Epidemiol Rec.* 2000 Jul 7;75(27):217-23

[46] *Venkataraman KS, Nedunchelliyan S.* Epidemiology of an outbreak of leptospirosis in man and dog. *Comp Immunol Microbiol Infect Dis.* 1992 Oct;15(4):243-7.

[47] *Srivastava DK.* Outbreak of Weil's disease in a food fad commune in India. *Br Med J (Clin Res Ed).* 1987 Apr 4;294(6576):905-6.

[48] *Singh KK.* Outbreak of Weil's disease in a food fad commune in India. *Br Med J (Clin Res Ed).* 1987 Feb 14;294(6569):443.

[49] *Agrawal PK, Srivastava DK.* Outbreak of Weil's disease in a food fad commune in India. *Br Med J (Clin Res Ed).* 1986 Dec 20-27;293(6562):1646-7.

[50] *Ratnam S, Sundararaj T, Subramanian S.* Serological evidence of leptospirosis in a human population following an outbreak of the disease in cattle. *Trans R Soc Trop Med Hyg*. 1983;77(1):94-8.

[51] *Mukherjea AK, Sen AK, Das AK, Mukherjee TP, Chatterjee BD, Mukherjee MK, Banik BG.* An outbreak of leptospirosis in Howrah, West Bengal. *Bull Calcutta Sch Trop Med.* 1972 Apr;20(2):26-7.

[52] *Tse KC, Yip PS, Hui KM, Li FK, Yuen KY, Lai KN, Chan TM.* Potential benefit of plasma exchange in treatment of severe icteric leptospirosis complicated by acute renal failure. *Clin Diagn Lab Immunol* 2002;9:482-4.

[53] Surachai N. New trends of treatment in Weil' disease : a case report 6/2 *Reg Med J* 1995; 2: 60-64.

[54] Phochanukul C, Sitprija V, Penchart C. Blood exchange in treatment of renal failure accompanied with jaundice in leptospirosis patients. *Chula Med J* 1973; 18: 99-103

[55] *Sitprija V, Chusilp S.* Renal failure and hyperbilirubinaemia in leptospirosis. Treatment with exchange transfusion. *Med J Aust.* 1973;1:171-3.

[56] *Pochanugool C, Sitprija V.* Hyperbilirubinemic renal failure in tropical disease: Treatment with exchange transfusion. *J Med Assoc* Thai. 1978 Jan;61 Suppl 1:75-7.

[57] *Niwattayakul K, Homvijitkul J, Khow O, Sitprija V.* Leptospirosis in northeastern Thailand: hypotension and complications. *Southeast Asian J Trop Med Public Health.* 2002;33:155-60.

[58] Wiwanitkit V. Comparison between blood exchange and classical therapy for acute renal failure in Weil's disease: appraisal on Thai reports. *Nephrology (Carlton*). 2006 Oct;11(5):481.

[59] Edwards CN, Levett PN. Prevention and treatment of leptospirosis. *Expert Rev Anti Infect Ther* 2004;2:293-8.

[60] Bharti AR, Nally JE, Ricaldi JN, Matthias MA, Diaz MM, Lovett MA, Levett PN, Gilman RH, Willig MR, Gotuzzo E, Vinetz JM; Peru-United States Leptospirosis Consortium. Leptospirosis: a zoonotic disease of global importance. *Lancet Infect Dis* 2003;3:757-71.

[61] Pappachan MJ, Sheela M, Aravindan KP. Relation of rainfall pattern and epidemic leptospirosis in the Indian state of Kerala. *J Epidemiol Community Health* 2004;58:1054 .

[62] Phraisuwan P, Whitney EA, Tharmaphornpilas P, Guharat S, Thongkamsamut S, Aresagig S, Liangphongphanthu J, Junthima K, Sokampang A, Ashford DA. Leptospirosis: skin wounds and control strategies, Thailand, 1999. *Emerg Infect Dis* 2002;8:1455-9.

[63] Kupek E, de Sousa Santos Faversani MC, de Souza Philippi JM. The relationship between rainfall and human leptospirosis in Florianopolis, Brazil, 1991-1996. *Braz J Infect Dis* 2000;4:131-4.

[64] Sejvar J, Tangkanakul W, Ratanasang P, Dowell SF, Sangjun N, Bragg S, Ashford D, Tappero J. An outbreak of leptospirosis, Thailand--the importance of the laboratory. *Southeast Asian J Trop Med Public Health* 2005;36:289-95.

Chapter III

Indian Malaria

Introduction to Malaria

Malaria is an important tropical mosquito-borne protozoa infection. It can be noted that malaria is a very important tropical mosquito-borne infectious disease affecting millions of the world's population annually. Malaria is caused by specific parasites of the genus Plasmodium. Five species of *Plasmodium*, *Plasmodium falciparum*, *Plasmodium vivax*, *Plasmodium ovale*, *Plasmodium malariae* and *Plasmodium knowlesii* can produce the human disease in its several forms. In humans, malaria is a potentially deadly mosquito-borne disease characterized by cyclical patterns of fever with severe myalgia, shaking and sweating found in the tropical countries [1 – 2]. Despite encouraging trends of decreasing malaria, the rates of the disease may be re-emerging in many tropical and non-tropical countries, especially in Asia, as evidence from an increased annual parasite index. Despite several years of malarial control success and a competent network of countrywide health infrastructure, malaria is still an important health threat in rural communities at present [3]. Members of 5 anopheline species complexes, *Anopheles dirus*, *Anopheles minimus*, *Anopheles sandicus*, *Anopheles aconitus* and *Anopheles manculatus*, registered to be primary malaria vectors, are also common in many tropical countries.

Although there have been many efforts for a long time to produce a vaccine to combat this infection, few have been able to meet the challenges harbored by the unusual interplay between this virus and human beings. Owing to present globalization, malaria becomes an emerging infectious problem not only to the tropical but also to the non-tropical countries in Europe and America. Angell and Cetron said that high-risk illnesses in travelers included malaria [4]. In addition, the problem of drug resistant malaria is significantly increasing. Wernsdorfer and Wernsdorfer noted that the drug resistance of malaria was the most common clinical problem in the fight against the disease since it affected the most elementary objective of malaria control, namely the elimination of mortality and the reduction of suffering from malaria [5]. The knowledge of malaria is, therefore, an interesting topic for clinicians.

Human beings can get the infection when a female vector mosquito injects a small, mobile form of the parasite, called a sporozoite, into the blood while having a meal. These sporozoites are then carried to the liver, where they will further reproduce [6 - 7]. By this process a single sporozoite eventually produces several thousand of what are called daughter merozoites, which discharge from burst liver cells into the blood and it is at this stage that the symptoms can be seen [6 - 7]. Once they are in the blood stream, the merozoites enter the erythrocytes, and therefore the parasite can then be seen in erythrocytes when they are examined under the standard light microscope [6 - 7]. Within the erythrocyte, further reproduction takes place and between 6 and 24 daughter merozoites are pushed out [6 - 7]. Each of these particles is capable of invading erythrocytes, and therefore the cycle is repeated [6 - 7]. Symptoms of malaria generally take around six days to be seen after infection [6 - 7]. Wide ranges of malarial symptoms are described in literature [6 - 7]. Some malarial patients complain of a headache, fatigue and muscle ache [6 - 7]. High fever is common, but these described symptoms are similar to a viral illness and can be mistaken for flu [6 - 7]. Some infected people presented with chest pain, abdominal pain, joint pains and diarrhea which imply something other than a viral illness [6 - 7].

Although there are many current advents in malarial diagnosis, most diagnoses in the endemic area are usually based on clinical history and basic screening tests done specifically for blood smear interpretation. There are two main blood smear preparation techniques for malarial investigation: thin film and thick film tests. Lee *et al* said that thin and thick blood film microscopy can be used as the gold standard for malaria diagnosis [8]. A thin blood smear is prepared based on a drop of blood that has been spread across a large area of the slide while a thick blood smear is a drop of blood on a glass slide [9]. Thin blood smears are most applicable in determining what species of malaria is causing the infection while thick blood smears are most applicable for detecting the presence of parasites, since they allow a larger sample of blood to be examined. Usually there are only a few parasites in the blood at the time the test is done [9].

The concept of malarial therapy is similar to other infections: getting rid of the pathogen or controlling the identified infection while providing supportive or symptomatic treatment. In malaria, many antimalarial drugs are in real clinical usage for a long time. The selection of anti-malarial drugs depends on the parasite species and the reported resistance pattern in each clinical setting [10]. Randomized controlled trials have not shown any significant benefit of the artemisinin derivatives over quinine in quinine sensitive areas [11]. Also, if quinine is given in the recommended way, the side effects are no better than artemisinins [11]. Drug resistance is a very important clinical problem in using anti-malarial drugs. Historically, the first case of chloroquine resistance was along the Thai-Cambodian border in the late 1950s; after that, Southeast Asia has played an important function as a focus for further development of drug resistance in *Plasmodium falciparum* [12]. In addition, the onset of chloroquine resistance marked the start of a new chapter in the history of malaria in Southeast Asia and by 1973 chloroquine finally had to be replaced by the combination of sulphadoxine and pyrimethamine as the first line drug for the therapy of uncomplicated malaria in Thailand. More than 10 African countries have also switched their first line drug to other newly developed antimalarial drugs [12]. In additional to specific malarial treatment, the supportive and symptomatic treatment is also clinically significant in taking care of malarial patients. Since several systemic complications like hypoglycemia, hypovolemia, hyperpyrexia, renal failure, bleeding disorders, anemia, lactic acidosis and pulmonary edema can lead to the pathogenesis of coma, and are responsible for high fatality, well designed supportive care along with intravenous administration of antimalarial drugs are the goals of malarial treatment [13].

The prevention of malaria is good means to control this parasitic disease. Since this disease is a vector-borne transmission, the control of the vector is very important in primary prevention of malaria. Bed nests and pesticides are widely used, aiming at primary prevention of malaria. Advances in prevention of malaria include new attempts to develop a vaccine and transgenic vectors for controlling this disease.

Indian Malaria

Malarial infection is the most prominent mosquito-borne disease. With an annual incidence of 300-500 million clinically diagnosed cases and a death toll of 1.1-2.7 million, malaria is a top communicable disease of the world [5]. Wernsdorfer and Wernsdorfer said that about 40% of the world's population live in areas where malaria is highly endemic [5]. They also noted that although this reflected the considerable effect of intensive malaria control, the disease continued to hit large populations in all parts of the tropics and subtropics [5]. Asia is the primary area of malaria cases. The endemic areas of malaria cover a wide range in the Asia region. South Asia also has the problem of malaria. In this chapter, the author uses the specific term of Indian malaria to describe the problem of malaria in South Asia.

1. Malaria in India

India is a big country. There are also some areas that lie in the tropical region. Therefore, the problem of malaria can be seen. The malaria can be classified as an important emerging infection in India [14]. There are many reports on emerging of malaria in India as shown in Table 1.

2. Malaria in Nepal

Nepal is another country in South Asia. There are no reports on the emergence of malaria in Nepal. This might be due to the fact that Nepal is not in the tropical area of Asia.

3. Malaria in Bhutan

Bhutan is another country in South Asia. There are no reports on the emergence of malaria in Bhutan. This might be due to the fact that Bhutan is not in the tropical area of Asia.

Table 1. Reports on the emergence of Malaria in India.

Author	Details
Das et al [15]	*Das et al reported on* malaria situation in forest-fringed villages of Sonitpur district of Assam, India bordering Arunachal Pradesh during an outbreak [15].
Borah et al [16]	*Borah* et al reported on clinical presentations of malaria during an out break situation in India [16].
Krishnamoorthy et al [17]	*Krishnamoorthy* et al reported on altered environment and risk of malaria outbreak in South Andaman, Andaman & Nicobar Islands, India affected by Asian tsunami disaster [17].
Singh et al [18]	*Singh* et al reproted an outbreak of malaria in a village in Faridabad district, Haryana, India [18].
Dev et al [19]	*Dev* et al reported an outbreak of Plasmodium falciparum malaria due to Anopheles minimus in central Assam, India [19].
Dhiman et al [20]	*Dhiman* et al reported on an investigation of malaria outbreak in Bahraich district, Uttar Pradesh, India [20].
Tyagi et al [21]	*Tyagi* et al reported on serological profile following malaria outbreak in Mewat region of Haryana, India [21].
Tyagi et al [22]	*Tyagi et al reported on* malaria outbreak in the Indira Gandhi Nahar Pariyojna command area in Jaisalmer district, Thar Desert, India [22].
Balaraman et al [23]	*Balaraman* et al reported on risk of outbreak of vector-borne diseases in the tsunami hit areas of southern India [23].
Ansari et al [24]	*Ansari et al reported on* epidemiologic investigations of a malaria outbreak in northern Delhi area, India [24].
Srivastava and Yada [25]	*Srivastava and Yadav* reported on malaria outbreak in a tribal area of Gujarat state, India [25].
Roy et al [26]	*Roy* et al reported on serological investigation of malaria outbreak in Thar desert of Rajasthan, India [26].
Prakash et al [27]	*Prakash* et al reported on epidemiology of malaria outbreak during, Apri and May, 1999, in Titabor Primary Health Centre, district Jorhat, Assam, India [27].
Mukhopadhyay [28]	*Mukhopadhyay* reported on malaria outbreak in 1997 in India [28].
Das et al [29]	Das et al reported on an epidemiological and entomological investigation on malaria outbreak at Tamulpur PHC, Assam, India [29].
Sharma et al [30]	*Sharma* et al reported on malaria outbreak in Mewat region Gurgaon district of Haryana State, india [30].
Bhuyan et al [31]	*Bhuyan* et al reported on the role of Anopheles culicifacies during an outbreak of malaria in Gorubandha P.H.C., Assam, India [31].
Sharma et al [32]	*Sharma* et al mentioned high prevalence of chloroquine resistant Plasmodium falciparum infection in Rajasthan epidemic [32].
Akhtar and McMichael [33]	*Akhtar and McMichael* reported on the correlation between rainfall and malaria outbreaks in western Rajasthan, India [33].
Prakash et al [34]	*Prakash* et al studied on vector incrimination in Tamulpur primary health centre, district Nalbari, lower Assam during malaria outbreak 1995 [34].

Mukhopadhyay [35]	*Mukhopadhyay* mentioned resurgence of malaria with special reference to malaria outbreak in Calcutta, India [35].
Bouma and van der Kaay [36]	*Bouma and van der Kaay* reported on the El Niño Southern Oscillation and the historic malaria epidemics on the Indian subcontinent and Sri Lanka [36]. They also raised the question of whether or not this was an early warning system for future epidemics [36].
Sharma [37]	*Sharma* reviewed and discussed the re-emergence of malaria in India [37].
Bouma and van der Kaay [38]	*Bouma and van der Kaay* reported on epidemic malaria in India's Thar desert [38].
Tyagi et al [39]	*Tyagi* et al reported on epidemic malaria in Thar desert, India [39].
Shukla et al [40]	*Shukla* et al reported on investigation of malaria outbreak in Rajasthan, India [40].
Adak et al [41]	*Adak* et al reported on an epidemiological study of malaria outbreak in a hotel construction site of Delhi, India [41].
Gupta and Kataria [42]	*Gupta and Kataria* reported on Plasmodium falciparum hepatitis during malaria epidemic in India [42].
Prasad et al [43]	*Prasad* et al reported on malaria epidemic in Baniyani village, District Farrukhabad (U.P.), India [43].
Mathur et al [44]	*Mathur* et al reported on epidemic of malaria in Barmer district (Thar desert) of Rajasthan during 1990 [44].
Sharma and Gautam [45]	*Sharma and Gautam* reported their studies on outbreak of malaria in Muliad village of Kheda district, Gujarat. , India [45]
Prasad and Sharma [46]	*Prasad and Sharma* reported on an outbreak of malaria in Banda PHC of District Shahjahanpur (U.P.). India [46].
Singh et al [47]	*Singh* et al reproted on malaria outbreak in Kundam block, district Jabalpur (M.P.). India [47].
Narasimham and Khamre [48]	*Narasimham and Khamre reported on* an epidemiological and entomological aspects of malaria outbreak during 1986-87 in Panaji, Goa [48].
Ansari et al [49]	*Ansari* et al reported on an outbreak of malaria in villages of Bareilly, District U.P. India [49].
Baukapur and Babu [50]	*Baukapur and Babu* reported on a focal outbreak of malaria in Valsad district, Gujarat State, India [50].
Ghosh et al [51]	*Ghosh* et al reported on an epidemiological and entomological features of an outbreak of fever in Meghraj Block, Sabarkantha District, Gujarat State (India) in 1980 [51].
Panicker et al [52]	*Panicker* et al wrote a note on an outbreak of malaria in Cuddalore, South Arcot district, Tamil Nadu. India [52].
Midha et al [53]	*Midha* et al reported on a focal outbreak of Plasmodium malariae infection in Rohtak District (Haryana). India [53]
Bhatt et al [54]	*Bhatt et* al reproted on a pre-monsoonic outbreak of malaria in the Khodiar Dam site labour colony. Amreli District, Saurashtra (Gujarat State), India [54].

4. Malaria in Maldives

Maldives is another country in South Asia. Of interest, there are no reports on the emergence of malaria in Maldives although this country lies in the tropical zone. This may be due to the fact that this country is a combination of several islands in the Indian ocean.

5. Malaria in Sri Lanka

Sri Lanka is another country in South Asia. Of interest, there are some reports on the emergence of malaria in Sri Lanka as presented in Table 2.

Table 2. Reports on the emergence of malaria in Sri Lanka.

Author	Details
Jones [55]	Jones reported on the Ceylon malaria epidemic of 1934-35 as a case study in colonial medicine [55].
Wijesundera et al [56]	*Wijesundera* et al studied on antibodies to Plasmodium falciparum sporozoites following a malarial outbreak in a non-endemic area of Sri Lanka [56].
Wijesundera Mde [57]	*Wijesundera Mde*_studied malaria outbreaks in new foci in Sri Lanka [57].
Sivagnanasundram [58]	*Sivagnanasundram*_studied reproduction rates of infection during the 1967-1968 Plasmodium vivax malaria epidemic in Sri Lanka [58].

6. Malaria in Bangladesh

Bangladesh is another country in South Asia. Of interest, there are some reports on the emergence of malaria in Bangladesh as presented in Table 3.

Table 3. Reports on the emergence of malaria in Bangladesh.

Author	Details
Maheswary et al [59]	Maheswary et al reported on incrimination of Anopheles aconitus Donitz as a vector of epidemic malaria in Bangladesh [59]
Maheswary et al [60]	Maheswary et al reported on incrimination of Anopheles vagus Donitz, 1902 as an epidemic malaria vector in Bangladesh [60].

7. Malaria in Pakistan

Pakistan is another country in South Asia. Of interest, there are some reports on the emergence of malaria in Pakistan as presented in Table 4.

Table 4. Reports on the emergence of malaria in Pakistan.

Author	Details
Bouma et al [61]	Bouma et al mentioned malaria control and long-term periodicity of the disease in Pakistan [61].
de Zulueta et al [62]	de Zulueta et al mentioned malaria control and long-term periodicity of the disease in Pakistan [62].

Pathology of Malaria

Several malarial pathological conditions are listed in the literature. The main alteration is on the erythrocyte as previously mentioned. The destruction of erythrocyte, owing to immunopathology, is proposed. Sherman *et al* noted that the human malaria parasite aged the erythrocyte during its intracellular development [63]. They said that during the stage of erythrocyte senescence the parasitized cell becomes less dense and deformable, its biconcave disc shape turns into a more spherical form and was covered with microscopic protuberances (knobs); the amounts of membrane cholesterol and phospholipids were disturbed and phosphatidylserine (PS) was externalized [63]. They noted that the malaria-infected cell is osmotically fragile, more permeable to a wide variety of particles by new permeation pathways (NPP), and there is superficial deposition of immunoglobulins and complement and there were declines in sialic acid, decreased glutathione, tocopherol and ATP [63]. They also mentioned that hemichromes were deposited on the inner side of the red cell membrane and there was clustering of the anion transporter, band 3 protein, as well as exposure of neoantigens, which contributed to antigenic variation and adhesivity of the parasitized erythrocyte [63]. Since erythrocyte carrying malarial parasites can travel thorough the bodies, the multisystemic pathological findings owing to malaria can be expected. Dondorp *et al* noted that autopsy studies, but also in vivo observations of the microcirculation, have shown variable obstructions of microcirculation in severe malaria [64]. They noted that the principal cause of this was cytoadherence to the vascular lining of erythrocytes containing the mature forms of the parasite, bringing sequestration and obstruction of small vessels [64]. In addition, they noted that parasitized erythrocytes turned rigid; compromising their flow through capillaries whose lumen had been reduced by sequestered erythrocytes [64]. They also mentioned that adhesive forces between malarial infected red cells (auto-agglutination), and uninfected red cells (rosetting) and between uninfected erythrocytes (aggregation) could further slow down microcirculatory flow and a more recent observation was that malarial infected erythrocytes also become rigid in severe malaria [64]. They finally proposed that reduction in the overall erythrocyte deformability has a strong predictive value for a deadly outcome [64].

Many complications of malaria are documented in literature. Rane *et al* said that there was an upward trend in deaths due to malaria and complications accounted for the majority of fatalities and cerebral malaria topped the list [65]. They noted that other complications detected were adult respiratory distress syndrome (ARDS), acute septicemic malaria, acute renal failure, (ARF) as well as disseminated intravascular coagulation (DIC) [65]. Concerning cerebral malaria, it is confirmed as the most serious complication. It is confirmed by sequestration of parasitized erythrocytes in cerebral capillaries and venules [66]. Mturi *et al* said that cerebral malaria was one of the most common nontraumatic encephalopathies at present [67]. Wassmer *et al* said that although the exact cause of cerebral malaria remained unclear, evidence had clearly implicated metabolic disturbances and its host immune responses [66]. They found that a greater accumulation of platelets occurred in capillaries and venules of the patients who died from cerebral malaria than from other conditions [66].

In addition to hematological pathology, the other rare clinical presentations of malaria are also documented. Hepatic manifestation is an important and rare presentation of malaria. The abnormality of the liver function test is also docmented in the literature. Recently, Wiwanitkit proposed that jaundice was not a rare presentation in the patients with malarial infection [68]. Yuda and Ishino said that malarial transmission to the human host was established by sporozoite infection of the hepatic and sporozoites are released from the mosquito salivary glands and flowed via blood stream to the hepatic sinusoid [69]. They noted that traversal of the sinusoidal cell layer and subsequent hepatic cell infection were the most important scenarios in sporozoite hepatic invasion, but the molecular basis of both events still needs to be elucidated [69]. They also said that this process was homologous to midgut epithelium penetration by the malarial ookinete, because identical genes were used in both processes [69]. Recent studies revealed that NKT cells participate in some types of hepatic injuries, especially for malaria hepatitis [70]. Malarial cirrhosis is an interesting complication of malarial infection. In 1981, Islam *et al* performed a clinical analysis of 293 cases of cirrhosis from two moderate-sized hospitals in Dacca and found that about one-tenth of the patients had past history of malaria [71]. Until recently, it can be said that there is an exact scenario for malarial hepatitis but the existence of malarial cirrhosis is still not confirmed [72 - 74]. However, Rothenberg *et al* stated that chronic liver diseases, especially cirrhosis, were not confirmed as exact late lesions of malaria [75]. The topic of malarial hepatitis is talked about a lot because it can be the presentation of the emergence of malaria which correlates with problematic hepatitis [68].

References

[1] Chareonviriyaphap T, Bangs MJ, Ratanatham S. Status of malaria in Thailand. *Southeast Asian J Trop Med. Public Health.* 2000; 31: 225-37.

[2] Phillips RS. Current status of malaria and potential for control. *Clin Microbiol.* 2001; 14: 208 – 26.

[3] Thimasarn K, Jatapadma S, Vijaykadga S, Sirichaisinthop J, Wongsrichanalai C. Epidemiology of Malaria in Thailand. *J Travel Med.* 1995; 2:59-65.

[4] Angell SY, Cetron MS. Health disparities among travelers visiting friends and relatives abroad. *Ann. Intern. Med.* 2005; 142: 67-72.

[5] Wernsdorfer G, Wernsdorfer WH. Malaria at the turn from the 2nd to the 3rd millenium. *Wien Klin Wochenschr.* 2003; 115 Suppl 3: 2-9.

[6] Suyaphun A, Wiwanitkit V, Suwansaksri J, Nithiuthai S, Sritar S, Suksirisampant W, Fongsungnern A. Malaria among hilltribe communities in northern Thailand: a review of clinical manifestations. *Southeast Asian J Trop Med Public Health.* 2002; 33 Suppl. 3: 14-5.

[7] Malaria. Available at http://www-micro.msb.le.ac.uk/224/Malaria.html

[8] Lee SH, Kara UA, Koay E, Lee MA, Lam S, Teo D. New strategies for the diagnosis and screening of malaria. *Int. J. Hematol.* 2002; 76 Suppl 1: 291-3.

[9] Thick and thin blood smears for malaria. Available at http://my.webmd.com/hw/health_guide_atoz/hw118744.asp

[10] Farooq U, Mahajan RC. Drug resistance in malaria. *J Vector Borne Dis.* 2004; 41: 45-53.

[11] Singhal T. Management of severe malaria. *Indian. J. Pediatr.* 2004; 71: 81-8.

[12] Indonesian Society of Medicine. *Consensus of Malaria Management* 2003 (part 2). Acta Med. Indones. 2004; 36: 187-93.

[13] Garg RK. Cerebral malaria. *J Assoc Physicians India.* 2000; 48: 1004-13.

[14] *Bhargava A, Chatterjee B.* Chikungunya fever, falciparum malaria, dengue fever, Japanese encephalitis... are we listening to the warning signs for public health in India? *Indian J Med Ethics.* 2007 Jan-Mar;4(1):18-23.

[15] *Das NG, Talukdar PK, Kalita J, Baruah I, Sribastava RB.* Malaria situation in forest-fringed villages of Sonitpur district (Assam), India bordering Arunachal Pradesh during an outbreak. J Vector Borne Dis. 2007 Sep;44(3):213-8.

[16] *Borah PK, Dutta P, Pegu P, Phukan AC, Hazarika NC, Mahanta J.* Clinical presentations of malaria during an out break situation. *J Commun Dis.* 2004 Mar;36(1):65-9.

[17] *Krishnamoorthy K, Jambulingam P, Natarajan R, Shriram AN, Das PK, Sehgal SC.* Altered environment and risk of malaria outbreak in South Andaman, Andaman & Nicobar Islands, India affected by tsunami disaster. *Malar J.* 2005 Jul 20;4:32.

[18] *Singh KB, Anand K, Krishna T, Kant S, Ray T, Kapoor SK.* An outbreak of malaria in a village in Faridabad district, Haryana. *Indian J Malariol.* 2000 Sep-Dec;37(3-4):106-10.

[19] *Dev V, Ansari MA, Hira CR, Barman K.* An outbreak of Plasmodium falciparum malaria due to Anopheles minimus in central Assam, India. *Indian J Malariol.* 2001 Mar-Jun;38(1-2):32-8.

[20] *Dhiman RC, Pillai CR, Subbarao SK.* Investigation of malaria outbreak in Bahraich district, Uttar Pradesh. *Indian J Med Res.* 2001 May;113:186-91.

[21] *Tyagi P, Roy A, Sreehari U, Ansari MA.* Serological profile following malaria outbreak in Mewat region of Haryana, India. *Indian J Malariol.* 2001 Sep-Dec;38(3-4):105-7.

[22] *Tyagi BK, Yadav SP, Sachdev R, Dam PK.* Malaria outbreak in the Indira Gandhi Nahar Pariyojna command area in Jaisalmer district, Thar Desert, *India. J Commun Dis.* 2001 Jun;33(2):88-95.

[23] *Balaraman K, Sabesan S, Jambulingam P, Gunasekaran K, Boopathi Doss PS.* Risk of outbreak of vector-borne diseases in the tsunami hit areas of southern India. *Lancet Infect Dis.* 2005 Mar;5(3):128-9.

[24] *Ansari MA, Sharma YD, Roy A, Biswas S, Sharma PK.* Epidemiologic investigations of a malaria outbreak in northern Delhi area. *J Am Mosq Control Assoc.* 2001 Dec;17(4):216-20.

[25] *Srivastava HC, Yadav RS.* Malaria outbreak in a tribal area of Gujarat state, India. *Southeast Asian J Trop Med Public Health.* 2000 Jun;31(2):219-24.

[26] *Roy A, Tyagi P, Biswas S.* Serological investigation of malaria outbreak in Thar desert of Rajasthan. *J Commun Dis.* 2000 Jun;32(2):123-8.

[27] *Prakash A, Mohapatra PK, Bhattacharyya DR, Sharma CK, Goswami BK, Hazarika NC, Mahanta J.* Epidemiology of malaria outbreak (April/May, 1999) in Titabor Primary Health Centre, district Jorhat (Assam). *Indian J Med Res.* 2000 Apr;111:121-6.

[28] *Mukhopadhyay SP.* Malaria outbreak 1997. *J Indian Med Assoc.* 1998 Nov;96(11):327, 329.

[29] *Das NG, Baruah I, Kamal S, Sarkar PK, Das SC, Santhanam K.* An epidemiological and entomological investigation on malaria outbreak at Tamulpur PHC, Assam. *Indian J Malariol.* 1997 Sep;34(3):164-70.

[30] *Sharma RS, Lal S, Sharma SN, Joshi RD, Dhillon GP.* Malaria outbreak in Mewat region Gurgaon district of Haryana State. *J Commun Dis.* 1997 Sep;29(3):307-8.

[31] *Bhuyan M, Das NG, Chakraborty BC, Talukdar PK, Sarkar PK, Das SC, Santhanam K.* Role of Anopheles culicifacies during an outbreak of malaria in Gorubandha P.H.C., Assam. *J Commun Dis.* 1997 Sep;29(3):243-6.

[32] *Sharma YD, Biswas S, Pillai CR, Ansari MA, Adak T, Devi CU.* High prevalence of chloroquine resistant Plasmodium falciparum infection in Rajasthan epidemic. *Acta Trop.* 1996 Dec 16;62(3):135-41.

[33] *Akhtar R, McMichael AJ.* Rainfall and malaria outbreaks in western Rajasthan. *Lancet.* 1996 Nov 23;348(9039):1457-8.

[34] *Prakash A, Mohapatra PK, Srivastava VK.* Vector incrimination in Tamulpur primary health centre, district Nalbari, lower Assam during malaria outbreak 1995. *Indian J Med Res.* 1996 Mar;103:146-9.

[35] *Mukhopadhyay SP.* Resurgence of malaria with special reference to malaria outbreak in Calcutta. *J Indian Med Assoc.* 1996 Apr;94(4):145-6.

[36] *Bouma MJ, van der Kaay HJ.* The El Niño Southern Oscillation and the historic malaria epidemics on the Indian subcontinent and Sri Lanka: an early warning system for future epidemics? *Trop Med Int Health.* 1996 Feb;1(1):86-96.

[37] *Sharma VP.* Re-emergence of malaria in India. *Indian J Med Res.* 1996 Jan;103:26-45.

[38] *Bouma MJ, van der Kaay.* Epidemic malaria in India's Thar desert. *Lancet.* 1995 Nov 4;346(8984):1232-3.

[39] *Tyagi BK, Chaudhary RC, Yadav SP.* Epidemic malaria in Thar desert, India. Lancet. 1995 Sep 2;346(8975):634-5.

[40] *Shukla RP, Pandey AC, Mathur A.* Investigation of malaria outbreak in Rajasthan. *Indian J Malariol.* 1995 Sep;32(3):119-28.

[41] *Adak T, Batra CP, Mittal PK, Sharma VP.* Epidemiological study of malaria outbreak in a hotel construction site of Delhi. *Indian J Malariol.* 1994 Sep;31(3):126-31.

[42] *Gupta UC, Kataria ML.* Plasmodium falciparum hepatitis during malaria epidemic. *J Assoc Physicians India.* 1993 May;41(5):292.

[43] *Prasad RN, Virk KJ, Sharma T, Dutta GD.* Malaria epidemic in Baniyani village, District Farrukhabad (U.P.). *Indian J Malariol.* 1992 Dec;29(4):219-24.

[44] *Mathur KK, Harpalani G, Kalra NL, Murthy GG, Narasimham MV.* Epidemic of malaria in Barmer district (Thar desert) of Rajasthan during 1990. *Indian J Malariol.* 1992 Mar;29(1):1-10.

[45] *Sharma RC, Gautam AS.* Studies on outbreak of malaria in Muliad village of Kheda district, Gujarat. *Indian J Malariol.* 1990 Sep;27(3):157-62.

[46] *Prasad RN, Sharma SN.* Outbreak of malaria in Banda PHC of District Shahjahanpur (U.P.). *Indian J Malariol.* 1990 Mar;27(1):47-50.

[47] *Singh N, Sharma VP, Shukla MM, Chand G.* Malaria outbreak in Kundam block, district Jabalpur (M.P.). *Indian J Malariol.* 1988 Jun;25(1):41-9

[48] *Narasimham MV, Khamre JS.* Epidemiological and entomological aspects of malaria outbreak during 1986-87 in Panaji, Goa. *J Commun Dis.* 1987 Jun;19(2):117-20.

[49] *Ansari MA, Batra CP, Sharma VP.* Outbreak of malaria in villages of Bareilly, District U.P. *Indian J Malariol.* 1984 Dec;21(2):121-3

[50] *Baukapur SN, Babu CJ.* A focal outbreak of malaria in Valsad district, Gujarat State. *J Commun Dis.* 1984 Dec;16(4):268-72.

[51] *Ghosh TK, Biswas S, Singh K, Dutta M, Bhardwaj M.* Epidemiological and entomological features of an outbreak of fever in Meghraj Block, Sabarkantha District, Gujarat State (India) in 1980. *J Commun Dis.* 1984 Sep;16(3):208-18.

[52] *Panicker KN, Chandrahas RK, Das PK.* Note on an outbreak of malaria in Cuddalore, South Arcot district, Tamil Nadu. *Indian J Med Res.* 1980 Jun;71:873-4.

[53] *Midha N, Grover PS, Sood VP, Chugh TD.* Focal outbreak of Plasmodium malariae infection in Rohtak District (Haryana). *Indian J Pathol Microbiol.* 1979 Oct;22(4):377.

[54] *Bhatt HR, Menon CP, Joshi TC.* A pre-monsoonic outbreak of malaria in the Khodiar Dam site labour colony. Amreli District, Saurashtra (Gujarat State), India. *Indian J Malariol.* 1962 Sep;16:215-21.

[55] Jones M. The Ceylon malaria epidemic of 1934-35: a case study in colonial medicine. *Soc Hist Med.* 2000 Apr;13(1):87-109.

[56] *Wijesundera MD, Peiris JS, Ariyaratne YG, Verdini AS, Pessi A, Del Giudice G.* Antibodies to Plasmodium falciparum sporozoites following a malarial outbreak in a non-endemic area of Sri Lanka. *Trans R Soc Trop Med Hyg.* 1990 Jan-Feb;84(1):35-9.

[57] *Wijesundera Mde S.* Malaria outbreaks in new foci in Sri Lanka. *Parasitol Today.* 1988 May;4(5):147-50.

[58] *Sivagnanasundram C.* Reproduction rates of infection during the 1967-1968 P. vivax malaria epidemic in Sri Lanka (Ceylon). *J Trop Med Hyg.* 1973 Apr;76(4):83-6.

[59] Maheswary NP, Majumdar S, Chowdhury AR, Faruque MS, Montanari RM. Incrimination of Anopheles aconitus Donitz as a vector of epidemic malaria in Bangladesh. *Southeast Asian J Trop Med Public Health.* 1992 Dec;23(4):798-801.

[60] Maheswary NP, Majumdar S, Chowdhury AR, Faruque MS, Montanari RM. Incrimination of Anopheles vagus Donitz, 1902 as an epidemic malaria vector in Bangladesh. *Indian J Malariol.* 1994 Mar;31(1):35-8.

[61] Bouma MJ, Dye C, van der Kaay HJ. Malaria control and long-term periodicity of the disease in Pakistan. *Trans R Soc Trop Med Hyg.* 1980;74(5):624-32.

[62] de Zulueta J, Mujtaba SM, Shah IH. Malaria control and long-term periodicity of the disease in Pakistan. *Trans R Soc Trop Med Hyg.* 1980;74(5):624-32.

[63] Sherman IW, Eda S, Winograd E. Erythrocyte aging and malaria. *Cell Mol. Biol.* (Noisy-le-grand). 2004; 50:159-69.

[64] Dondorp AM, Pongponratn E, White NJ. Reduced microcirculatory flow in severe falciparum malaria: pathophysiology and electron-microscopic pathology. *Acta Trop.* 2004;89:309-17.

[65] Rane SR, Bapat VM, Holla W. Malaria still a threat to life--a postmortem study. *Indian J. Pathol. Microbiol.* 2003; 46: 17-9.

[66] Wassmer SC, Coltel N, Combes V, Grau GE. Pathogenesis of cerebral malaria: facts and hypotheses. *Med. Trop. (Mars*). 2003; 63: 254-7.

[67] Mturi N, Musumba CO, Wamola BM, Ogutu BR, Newton CR. Cerebral malaria: optimising management. CNS. *Drugs.* 2003; 17: 153-65.

[68] Wiwanitkit V. Jaundice as co-presentation in Thai malarial patients. *J Indian Med* Assoc. 2004; 102: 107.

[69] Yuda M, Ishino T. Liver invasion by malarial parasites--how do malarial parasites break through the host barrier? *Cell Microbiol.* 2004; 6:1119-25.

[70] Tsutsui H, Adachi K, Seki E, Nakanishi K. Cytokine-induced inflammatory liver injuries. *Curr Mol Med.* 2003; 3: 545-59.

[71] Islam N, Khan M, Ahmed Z. Cirrhosis of liver. *Bangladesh Med Res. Counc. Bull.* 1981; 7: 45-51.

[72] Mahi PN, Tandon HD. Malarial hepatitis. *J. Indiana State Med Assoc.* 1955; 25 : 507-11.

[73] Gyergyay F, Hermann E. Etiopathogenetic factors in liver cirrhosis. *Med Interna* (Bucur). 1956; 8: 669-79.

[74] Franken HF, Snoos A. Is there a malaria cirrhosis? *Munch Med Wochenschr.* 1996; 108: 879-83.

[75] Rothenberg G, Schubert S. Assessment of late complications of malaria in travelers to the tropics. *Z. Gesamte Inn Med.* 1983; 38: 46-7.

Chapter IV

Leishmaniasis in India

Introduction to Leishmaniasis

Leishmaniasis is an important tropical vector-borne infection. There are two main forms of leishmaniasis, the cutaneous and visceral forms. Leishmanioses are a group of blood parasitic diseases that affect man and also other mammals. The infections are caused by different species of trypanosomatids of the genus Leishmania [1 – 2]. Leishmaniasis is confirmed as a complex of diseases with a clinical and epidemiological diversity [3]. Leishmaniasis is still a severe public health problem and its burden is increasing in many countries [3]. As already mentioned, this disease is generated by a parasite belonging to the genus Leishmania [3]. Approximately 350 billion people in 88 different countries are noted to be infected with this parasite [3]. The distribution of this re-emerging disease, which is found throughout the world, is believed to be due to various factors linked to both human activity and climatic change [2]. The heteroecious life cycle of this blood parasite includes an invertebrate host (sandflies of the Phlebotomidae family) [2 - 4]. The dog is the main carrier of this disease [2 – 4].

Based on parasite and host factors and immunoinflammatory responses, the clinical presentation of this blood infection includes subclinical (inapparent), localised (skin lesions), and disseminated infection (cutaneous, mucosal, or visceral) [5]. Symptomatic disease is a subacute or chronic disease and has many forms of presentation and outcome [5]. Cutaneous leishmaniasis and VL are the two main forms of leishmaniasis as previously noted. Leishmania species, present both cutaneous and visceral clinical signs and symptoms [2 - 4]. Visceral leishmaniases (VL), with spreading epidemics in India, and sporadic cases in the mediterranean basin, show clinical, therapeutical and public health aspects varying in accordance to specific geographic context [6]. VL is classified an important fatal tropical blood infection.

VL is of higher priority than cutaneous leishmaniasis as it is a deadly disease and has no good treatment [7]. Anthroponotic VL foci are of special consideration as they are found at the origin of the epidemics [7]. The leishmaniasis burden is still presently important: 350 million people are at risk, 500,000 new infected cases of VL annually, 1-1.5 million of cutaneous leishmaniasis: 2.4 millions [7]. Most of the burden is concentrated on few specific countries which show clear geographic priorities [7]. Leishmaniasis is still an important public health problem owing to not only environmental risk factors such as massive migrations, urbanisation, deforestation, and new irrigation schemes, but also to individual risk factors which include HIV, malnutrition, genetics, etc [7]. The extent and presentation of this blood infectious disease depends on several factors, including the humoral and cell-mediated immune response of the host, the virulence of the infecting species, and the parasite burden [8]. Children have proved to be at greater risk than adults in endemic areas. Malnutrition contributes to the development of disease, and incomplete medical therapy of leishmaniasis is a risk factor for recurrence of leishmaniasis [8]. Molecular methods can offer the promise of accurate non-invasive investigations for the diagnosis of this disease [8]. Globally, with the notable exception of India, pentavalent antimonial compounds remain the most effective and the most affordable medical therapy for leishmaniasis [8]. Lipid formulations of amphotericin B were assessed as short duration treatment and were confirmed to be effective [8]. However, their cost prohibited their wide use in several developing countries [8].

Leishmaniais in India

Leishmainal infection is an important vector-borne disease. With an annual incidence of millions of clinically diagnosed cases, this disease is still one of the main communicable diseases in the world [9 – 11]. This reflects a need for intensive leishmanial control because the disease still continues to hit large populations in all parts of the tropics and subtropics [9 - 11]. Asia is an area of leishmaniasis. The endemic areas of leishmaniasis cover some specific area of the Asian region. South Asia is a specific area that has confirmed having the problem of leishmaniasis. In this chapter, the author uses the specific term of Indian leishmaniasis to describe the problem of leishmaniasis in the South Asia.

1. Leishmaniasis in India

India is a big country. There are also some areas that lie in the tropical region. Therefore, the problem of leishmaniasis can be seen. The leishmaniasis can be classified as an important emerging infection in India. There are many reports on the emergence of leishmaniasis in India as shown in Table 1.

2. Leishmaniasis in Nepal

Nepal is another country in South Asia. There are no reports on the emergence of leishmaniasis in Nepal. This might be due to the fact that Nepal is not in the tropical area of Asia.

Table 1. Reports on the emergence of leishmaniasis in India.

Author	Details
Sharma et al [9]	Sharma et al reported on a re-emergence of visceral leishmaniasis in Gujarat, India [9].
Verma et al [10]	Verma et al reported on the observation of sodium stibogluconate-sensitive visceral leishmaniasis in the non-endemic hilly region of Uttarakhand, India [10].
Mathur et al [11]	Mathur et al reported on visceral leishmaniasis/human immunodeficiency virus co-infection in India observed in the focus of two epidemics [11].
Sundar et al [12]	Sundar et al reported on failure of pentavalent antimony in visceral leishmaniasis from the center of the Indian epidemic [12].
Kumar et al [13]	Kumar et al reported on a kala-azar epidemic in Varanasi district, India [13].
Bhatia et al [14]	Bhatia et al reported on an outbreak of kala-azar in Bombay [14].
Pathare [15]	Pathare raised the question "Is there an endemic focus of kala azar in Bombay?" in 1994 [15]
Addy and Nandy [16]	Addy and Nandy reported on the scenario of ten years of kala-azar in west Bengal and raised the question "Did post-kala-azar dermal leishmaniasis initiate the outbreak in Parganas?" [15]
Grover [17]	Grover noted on the resurgence of Kala-azar in India [17].
Rai et al [18]	Rai et al reported on clinico-epidemiological profiles of post-kala-azar dermal leishmaniasis in Varanasi, India [18].
Saxena [19]	Saxena studied collected sandflies from a kala-azar outbreak area of district Darbhanga (Bihar), India [19].
Chakraborty [20]	Chakraborty et al reported on outbreaks of kala-azar in Malda and Murshidabad districts of West Bengal, India [20].

3. Leishmaniasis in Bhutan

Bhutan is another country in South Asia. There are no reports on the emergence of leishmaniasis in Bhutan. This might be due to the fact that Bhutan is not in the tropical area of Asia.

4. Leishmaniasis in Maldives

Maldives is another country in South Asia. Of interest, there are no reports on the emergence of leishmaniasis in Maldives although this country lies in tropical zone. This may be due to the fact that this country is a combination of several islands in the Indian ocean.

5. Leishmaniasis in Sri Lanka

Sri Lanka is another country in South Asia. However, there is no report on outbreaks or epidemics of leishmaniasis in Sri Lanka.

6. Leishmaniasis in Bangladesh

Bangladesh is another country in South Asia. However, there is no report on outbreaks or epidemics of leishmaniasis in Bangladesh.

7. Leishmaniasis in Pakistan

Pakistan is another country in South Asia. However, there is no report on outbreaks or epidemics of leishmaniasis in Pakistan.

Diagnosis, Treatment and Prevention of Leishmaniasis at Present

For VL, diagnosis is mainly by determination of the parasite in bone marrow specimens (several biopsies are often required) or in the spleen [21]. The diagnosis of VL is hardly from the lymph nodes, or the hepatic tissues [22]. Bacteriologic studies using a special medium can be applicable [21]. Serologic tests are sensitive and specific but often give positivity only in late VL [21]. Cultures can be done on NNN medium, a biphasic medium, or liquid media with fetal calf serum [23]. The blood parasite demonstration and isolation rates are rather poor from cutaneous and mucocutaneous lesions due to low parasite load and high rate of contamination in microbiological culture [22]. Serologic testing is helpful with the indirect fluorescent antibody test (IFAT), [23]. However, IFAT can have cross-reactivity in patients who have leprosy, tuberculosis, malaria, schistosomiasis, Chagas disease, and African trypanosomiasis [23]. ELISA methods are also available. Recently, several recombinant proteins have been developed to help the diagnosis of VL. Recombinant kinesin protein of 39 kDa, called rK 39, is widely discussed at present. The antigen used in several test forms has been proved highly sensitive and specific for VL [23]. It is helpful in the diagnosis of HIV-Leishmania co-infection and can be used as a possible prognostic marker [23]. With the recent advances in medical biology, PCR methods were also launched for helping diagnosis of VL [24]. For cutaneous leishmaniasis, direct microscopic examination is helpful for diagnosis. Patients commonly have a single ulcer that can heal spontaneously, therefore, they require only topical, or no treatment at all [25]. Traditional diagnostic investigations for individual cases search for suggestive history and clinical features, the identification of amastigotes by histology or direct microscopy, and the growth of promastigotes in specific microbiological culture [26]. Diagnosis by the PCR seems to be a new gold standard and is widely applied as a novel technique, offering considerable advantages in the collection and transport of specimens and DNA extraction procedures that are more effective in individual and field-based works [26]. Several reports show up to 100% specificity with increasing sensitivity that overall is between 92 and 98% [26].

Considering therapy, medical therapy is the tract for treament. For VL, pentavalent antimonials (Sbv) have been effectively used for treatment of kala-azar for years [27 - 28]. Pentavalent antimonials are the first-line treatment options worldwide; however, there exists the problem of resistance to this drug in India [29]. The therapeutic regimen for VL is currently obstructed by several limitations as the available drugs are usually toxic. In addition, drug administrations are effective only parenterally and need to be administered for extended periods [28]. Recently, miltefosine (hexadecylphosphocholine), a compound originally developed as an antitumour agent has been shown to be an orally effective drug against kala-azar and was proposed as a new alternative for VL [30]. The first orally effective drug, miltefosine, has been presently approved [30]. In antimony refractory zones, amphotericin B deoxycholate is indicated, but prolonged hospitalization, toxic effects, and requirement for monitoring greatly hamper its widespread application in endemic regions [31]. Lipid formulations of amphotericin B, a remarkable advance in amphotericin B therapy, can help decrease toxicity and this enables large doses to be delivered over a short period [31]. Amphotericin B deoxycholate is the drug of choice in India at present [30]. It should be noted that although liposomal amphotericin B is the best antileishmanial formulation, its prohibitive cost prevents its use in endemic areas [30]. The combination of the two most potent leishmanicidal drugs amphotericin B and miltefosine, which are not dependent on host immune system, may shorten the course of therapy and should be preferred when treating kala-azar associated with HIV [32]. For cutaneous leishmaniasis, local treatment includes topical paromomycin, cryotherapy, localized controlled heat, carbon dioxide laser therapy, or intralesional meglumine antimoniate. Oral fluconazole may be selected as a second-line treatment. Parenteral antimonials are still helpful for persistent or recurrent Old World leishmaniasis [31. For New World leishmaniasis, parenteral antimonials represent the first-line treatment in all forms except those caused by Leishmania guyanensis in which pentamidine is more effective [31]. The success of treatment of cutaneous leishmaniasis should be assessed one and a half months after it has been completed and patients should be followed up for a half year [31].

For prevention of leishmaniasis, the vector control principle is applicable since this disease is a vector-borne disease [32 - 33]. Interruption of the pathway of infection by vector control can bring a cheaper, more practical solution to treatment and improved knowledge of the alternatives available could lead to preventative measures [33]. Different means to control phlebotomine sandflies, including residual spraying of dwellings and animal shelters, insecticide treated nets, application of repellents/insecticides to skin or to fabrics and impregnated dog collars are discussed in literature [33]. Indoor residual spraying is a simple and cost effective method of controlling endophilic vectors and DDT remains the insecticide of choice for the control of this disease [32]. However resistance to insecticide is likely to become more widespread in the population especially in those areas in which insecticide has been used for a long time [32]. In this context, use of slow-release emulsified suspension can be the best alternative. It is also noted that DDT resistant *P. argentipes*, particularly in endemic zones, is rapidly increasinng [34]. Although effective in urban areas with high concentrations of sandflies, residual spraying of insecticides is no longer tenable in most cases. The role of biological control and environment management in the control of leishmaniasis has been mentioned [32]. Allethrin (coil) 0.1 and 1.6 per cent prallethrin (liquid) have been found to be effective repellents against the insect vector of kala azar in India [32]. Insecticide impregnated bednets is another areas needs further research on priority basis for the control of this disease [32]. Vaccine for leishmaniasis is the new means for prevention. Searching for the leishmaniasis vaccine is the focused research point at present [35]. Candidates, including live or killed parasites, Leishmania purified fractions, defined recombinant parasite antigens, live recombinant bacteria expressing Leishmania antigens and antigen-encoding DNA plasmids, are presently being researched and developed [36].

Leishmaniasis in Areas Nearby to India

To help the reader more understand of the situation of leishmaniasis, the author hereby will discuss on the situation of leishmanisis in other nearby areas of India including the Middle East, the area to the right of India, Southeast Asia, and the area to the left of India.

A. Leishmaniasis in Southeast Asia

Leishmaniasis is not an endemic disease in Southeast Asia. There are no reports on the outbreak of leishmaniasis in Southeast Asia. The cases are usually sporadic. To help the reader better understand, the author hereby will present a small research on leishmaniasis in Southeast Asia using Thailand as a model.

Introduction

VL, with spreading epidemics in India, and sporadic cases in the mediterranean basin, show clinical, therapeutical and public health aspects varying according to the geographic context, therefore, it is useul to study the scenario of VL, an important tropical blood infection, in other settings. Although Thailand has high prevalence of the vector-borne diseases malaria and dengue fever, the VL is a non-endemic infectious disease and is rarely reported. In Thailand, the first case report of leishmaniasis infection was published in 1981 by Puavilai et al [37]. Since the first case report, there have been sporadic case reports of leishmaniasis in Thailand. Most of the cases are classified as being in the cutaneous form.

Here, the author performed a literature review of the reports of bone marrow leishmaniasis in Thailand in order to summarize the characteristics of this infection among Thai patients.

Materials and Methods

This study was designed as a descriptive retrospective study. A literature review of the papers concerning bone marrow leishmaniasis in Thailand was performed, using the database of published works cited in the Index Medicus and Science Citation Index. The author also reviewed the published works in all 256 local Thai journals, which are not included in the international citation index. The literature review focused on the years 1981 - 2005. The key word for searching was "lesimaniasis." According to the literature review, there were 23 reports on lesihmaniasis. Of these, 4 reports of bone marrow leishmaniasis were used for further study. The details of clinical presentations of the patients (such as clinical manifestation, diagnosis, treatment, and discharge status) were all included in the reports that were studied. The demographic data of all cases, including age and sex, were reviewed as well. Descriptive statistics were used in analyzing the patient characteristics. All the statistical analyses in this study were made using SPSS 7.0 for Windows.

Results

According to this study, there have been at least 4 reports [38 - 41] in the literature of 5 cases of bone marrow leishmaniasis in the Thai population, of which no case was lethal. Of all 5 cases, 4 were males and 1 was female. The average age was between 23.3 and 15.2 years old. No cases were immunocompromised. Concerning the clinical manifestations, all except one had prolonged fever with unknown origin. From physical examination, all had hepatosplenomegaly. At the time of diagnosis, peripheral blood smear could not demonstrate the parasites. But pancytopenia could be seen in all cases. The bone marrow study was performed and revealed increased bone marrow cellularity, adequate production of magakaryocytes, erythroid and myeloid precursors. The striking findings were active hemophagocytosis with increased proliferation of lymphoidplasma cell line in the bone marrow, and amastigotes of Leishmania donovani was demonstrated. Considering the treatment, pantavalent antimony compound was used and the excellent improvement and complete recovery of the clinical and hematologic abnormalities were obtained promptly after the administration.

Discussion

As already mentioned earlier, the distribution of re-emerging forms of the disease can be found throughout the world (except in Antarctica) and is influenced by various factors linked to both human activity and climatic change. The heteroecious life cycle of the Leishmania includes an invertebrate host or vector insects [2 - 4]. The dog is the main carrier for many of the Leishmania species, simultaneously presenting both cutaneous and visceral clinical signs [2 – 4]. Considering VL, the typical symptomatic triad, anemia-fever-enlarged spleen, may not be fully complete. The diagnosis of the visceral form is conventionally performed by the demonstration of amastigotes of this specific blood parasite in the aspirated fluid from the bone marrow, the spleen, sometimes from the lymph nodes, or the liver [5]. Berentsen et al said that the identification of the parasites in bone marrow biopsy should be performed in pancytopenic patients in patients of unknown origin who had history of visiting the Mediteranian, the endemic area of VL [42]. According to this study, it can be seen that all bone marrow leishmaniasis cases had a history of visiting the Middle East. All had the classical triads but smears revealed no organisms. Indeed, in Thailand, other tropical infectious diseases such as malaria can give the picture of triad as well. However, the bone marrow aspiration used to find the cause of unexplained pancytopenia can bring the final diagnoses in all cases [42]. Of interest, the author did not see the case that got the infection from India, which is the nearer endemic area of disease.

In this series, the bone marrow appearance show classical findings according to the bone marrow leishmaniasis. Detection of amastigote is the hallmark of diagnosis. However, some other rare appearances such as myelofibrosis are also reported [43]. Concerning the treatment, the pantavalent antimony is effective. Complete cure can be derived in all cases in this series. For treating VL, pentavalent antimonial compounds can still be the first-line agents in Thailand. However, due to trends of increasing resistance to this agent, many infected patients at present require other drugs including amphotericin B and pentamidine. Indeed, reported toxic effects of these second-line agents have brought new development of drug delivery systems like liposomal amphotericin B, which has demonstrated uniform efficacy in clinical trials [44].

B. Leishmaniasis in Middle East

Leishmaniasis is very common in Middle East. It can be said that the Middle East is the world endemic area of leishmaniasis [45 – 48]. A number of outbreaks of leishmaniasis are reported from the Middle East (Table 2).

In summary, it can be seen that the areas left of India (the Middle East) has endemicity of leishmaniasis. The disease is very common, whereas the disease exists in some specific parts of India, especially those next to the Middle East. Considering Southeast Asia, the disease is only sporadic and imported from the endemic area of Middle East. This can show that India is the buffer area between highly endemic area and an area free of disease. The vector distribution might be the answer to this scenario.

Table 2. Reports on the emergence of leishmaniasis in Middle East.

Author	Details
Faulde et al [49]	*Faulde* et al reported on zoonotic cutaneous leishmaniasis outbreak in Mazar-e Sharif, northern Afghanistan by mean of an epidemiological evaluation [49].
Leslie et al [50]	*Leslie et al reported on outbreak of* VL in Afghanistan [50].
Nasereddin et al [51]	*Nasereddin* et al mentioned for molecular fingerprinting of Leishmania infantum strains following an outbreak of VL in central Israel [51].
Yaghoobi-Ershadi et al [52]	*Yaghoobi-Ershadi et* al reported on a new epidemic focus of zoonotic cutaneous leishmaniasis in central Iran [52].
Reithinger et al [53]	*Reithinger* et al reported on cutaneous leishmaniasis, northern Afghanistan [53].
Reyburn et al [54]	*Reyburn* et al reported on the prolonged epidemic of anthroponotic cutaneous leishmaniasis in Kabul, Afghanistan [54].
Jacobson et al [55]	*Jacobson* et al reported on an outbreak of cutaneous leishmaniasis in northern northern Israel [55].
Yaghoobi-Ershadi et al [56]	*Yaghoobi-Ershadi et al reported on* a new focus of cutaneous leishmaniasis caused by *Leishmania tropica* in Middle East [56]
Volf et al [57]	*Volf* et al studied on sand flies in Sanliurfa, Turkey for the relationship of *Phlebotomus sergenti* with the epidemic of anthroponotic cutaneous leishmaniasis [57].
Yaghoobi-Ershadi et al [58]	*Yaghoobi-Ershadi et* al performed an epidemiological study in a new focus of cutaneous leishmaniosis due to Leishmania major in Ardestan town, central Iran [58].
Khoury et al [59]	*Khoury et al reported on an* outbreak of cutaneous leishmaniasis in a nonimmune population of soldiers in Wadi Araba, Jordan [59].
Alptekin et al [60]	*Alptekin et* al reported that sandflies associated with epidemic cutaneous leishmaniasis in Sanliurfa, Turkey [60].
Tayeh et al [61]	*Tayeh* et al summaried on the experience from 20 years of cutaneous leishmaniasis in Aleppo, Syria [61].
Jumaian et al [62]	*Jumaian* et al reported on an outbreak of cutaneous leishmaniasis in a nonimmune population of soldiers in Wadi Araba, Jordan [62].
Gramiccia et al [63]	*Gramiccia* et al reported on isoenzyme characterization of Leishmania isolates from human cases of cutaneous leishmaniasis in Urfa, south-east Turkey [63].
Büttiker and Lewis [64]	*Büttiker and Lewis* studied on ecological studies at Hofuf, Eastern Saudi Arabia, in relation to dermal leishmaniasis [64].
Nadim et al [65]	*Nadim* et al reported on situation of cutaneous leishmaniasis in Saudi-Arabia [65].
Koufman and Egoz [66]	*Koufman and Egoz* reported that Nebi Mussa was a new focus of cutaneous leishmaniasis in Middle East [66].

References

[1] Murray HW, Berman JD, Davies CR, Saravia NG. Advances in leishmaniasis. *Lancet.* 2005;366:1561-77

[2] Gallego M. Emerging parasitic zoonoses: leishmaniosis, *Rev. Sci. Tech.* 2004;23:661-76.

[3] Yurdakul P. Immunopathogenesis of Leishmania infections. *Mikrobiyol. Bul.* 2005;39:363-81.
[4] Piscopo TV, Mallia AC. Leishmaniasis. *Postgrad. Med. J.* 2006;82:649-57
[5] Murray HW, Berman JD, Davies CR, Saravia NG. Advances in leishmaniasis. *Lancet.* 2005;366:1561-77
[6] Rosenthal E, Marty P. Visceral leishmaniases. *Rev. Prat.* 2004;54:2211-6
[7] Desjeux P. Leishmaniasis: current situation and new perspectives. *Comp. Immunol. Microbiol. Infect. Dis.* 2004;27:305-18.
[8] Kafetzis DA. An overview of paediatric leishmaniasis. *J. Postgrad. Med.* 2003;49:31-8.
[9] Sharma U, Redhu NS, Mathur P, Singh S. Re-emergence of visceral leishmaniasis in Gujarat, India. *J Vector Borne Dis.* 2007 Sep;44(3):230-2.
[10] Verma SK, Ahmad S, Shirazi N, Kusum A, Kaushik RM, Barthwal SP. Sodium stibogluconate-sensitive visceral leishmaniasis in the non-endemic hilly region of Uttarakhand, India. *Trans R Soc Trop Med Hyg.* 2007 Jul;101(7):730-2.
[11] Mathur P, Samantaray JC, Vajpayee M, Samanta P. Visceral leishmaniasis/human immunodeficiency virus co-infection in India: the focus of two epidemics. *J Med Microbiol.* 2006 Jul;55(Pt 7):919-22.
[12] Sundar S, More DK, Singh MK, Singh VP, Sharma S, Makharia A, Kumar PC, Murray HW. Failure of pentavalent antimony in visceral leishmaniasis in India: report from the center of the Indian epidemic. *Clin Infect Dis.* 2000 Oct;31(4):1104-7.
[13] Kumar R, Kumar P, Chowdhary RK, Pai K, Mishra CP, Kumar K, Pandey HP, Singh VP, Sundar S. Kala-azar epidemic in Varanasi district, India. *Bull World Health Organ.* 1999;77(5):371-4.
[14] Bhatia S, Patel N, Gulhane S, Dongre V, Jijina FF, Pathare AV. Outbreak of kala-azar in Bombay. *J Postgrad Med.* 1995 Jan-Mar;41(1):3-4.
[15] Pathare AV. Is there an endemic focus of kala azar in Bombay? *J Postgrad Med.* 1994 Apr-Jun;40(2):55-6.
[16] Addy M, Nandy A. Ten years of kala-azar in west Bengal, Part I. Did post-kala-azar dermal leishmaniasis initiate the outbreak in 24-Parganas? *Bull World Health Organ.* 1992;70(3):341-6.
[17] Grover NK. Kala-azar--a resurgence. *J Indian Med Assoc.* 1991 Dec;89(12):329-30
[18] Rai RN, Kumar M, Srivastava A, Joshi RD, Asthana AK, Tripathi VC, Dutta KK. Clinico-epidemiological profiles of post-kala-azar dermal leishmaniasis in Varanasi. *J Commun Dis.* 1989 Sep;21(3):214-7.
[19] Saxena VK. Sandflies from a kala-azar outbreak area of district Darbhanga (Bihar), India. *J Commun Dis.* 1987 Dec;19(4):405-7
[20] Chakraborty S, Dutta M, Srivastava L, Barui KC, Mandal SP. Current outbreaks of kala-azar in Malda and Murshidabad districts of West Bengal--an epidemiological evaluation. *J Commun Dis.* 1982 Dec;14(4):263-73.
[21] Lagardere B, Chevallier B, Cheriet R. Kala-azar. *Ann. Pediatr. (Paris).* 1992;39:159-64.
[22] Singh S, Sivakumar R. Recent advances in the diagnosis of leishmaniasis. *J. Postgrad. Med.* 2003;49:55-60.
[23] Leishmaniasis. Available online at http://www.emedicine.com/emerg/topic296.htm

[24] Mortarino M, Franceschi A, Mancianti F, Bazzocchi C, Genchi C, Bandi C. Quantitative PCR in the diagnosis of Leishmania] *Parassitologia.* 2004;46:163-7.

[25] Hepbum NC. Cutaneous leishmaniasis: an overview. J. Postgrad. Med. 2003;49:50-4.

[26] Vega-Lopez F. Diagnosis of cutaneous leishmaniasis. *Curr. Opin. Infect. Dis.* 2003;16:97-101.

[27] Jha TK. Drug unresponsiveness and combination therapy for kala-azar. *Indian J. Med. Res.* 2006;123:389-98.

[28] Sundar S, Chatterjee M. Visceral leishmaniasis - current therapeutic modalities. *Indian J. Med. Res.* 2006;123:345-52.

[29] Sundar S, Rai M. Treatment of visceral leishmaniasis. Expert Opin. *Pharmacother.* 2005;6:2821-9.

[30] Sangraula H, Sharma KK, Rijal S, Dwivedi S, Koirala S. Orally effective drugs for kala-azar (visceral leishmaniasis): focus on miltefosine and sitamaquine. *J. Assoc. Physicians India.* 2003;51:686-90.

[31] Minodier P, Noel G, Blanc P, Uters M, Retornaz K, Garnier JM. Management of cutaneous leishmaniasis in adults and children. *Med. Trop. (Mars).* 2005;65:487-95.

[32] Kishore K, Kumar V, Kesari S, Dinesh DS, Kumar AJ, Das P, Bhattacharya SK. Vector control in leishmaniasis. *Indian J. Med. Res.* 2006;123:467-72.

[33] Maroli M, Khoury C. Prevention and control of leishmaniasis vectors: current approaches. *Parassitologia.* 2004;46:211-5.

[34] Kishore K, Kumar V, Kesari S, Bhattacharya SK, Das P. Susceptibility of Phlebotomus argentipes against DDT in endemic Districts of North Bihar, *India. J. Commun. Dis.* 2004;36:41-4.

[35] Poot J. Search for a vaccine against leishmaniasis] Tijdschr Diergeneeskd. 2006;131:694-5.

[36] Gradoni L. An update on antileishmanial vaccine candidates and prospects for a canine Leishmania vaccine. *Vet. Parasitol.* 2001;100:87-103.

[37] Puavilai S, Sirinavin S, Chirachariyavej T. Cutaneous leishmaniasis: report of a case. *Ramathibodi Med J* 1981; 4: 179 – 83.

[38] Chutaputti A, Siripool P, Chitchang S, Radomyos P. Visceral leishmaniasis (Kala-azar): with hypersplenism successfully treated with pentavalent antimony : report of 2 cases. *Intern Med* 1986; 2: 262 – 5

[39] Chutaputhi A, Siripool P, Chitchang S, Radomyos P. Visceral leishmaniasis (Kala-azar): a case report. *R Thai Army Med J* 1986; 39: 98 – 5

[40] Seksarn P, Chumdermpadetsuk S, Dharmkrong-At A, Likitnukul S, Mitrakul C, Poshyachinda M. Visceral leishmaniasis: a case report. *Chula Med J* 1984; 28: 1161-1170

[41] Tantaterdtham S, Susaengrat W. Visceral leishmaniasis : a case report (from Khon Kaen Regional Hospital). *J Infect Dis Antimicrob Agents* 1991; 8 : 161-163.

[42] Berentsen S, Langholm R, Reitan O. Visceral leishmaniasis (kala-azar). Tidsskr Nor Laegeforen. 1990;110:3491-3.

[43] Suvajdzic N, Pavlovic M, Misic S, Cemerikic V, Atkinson HD, Colovic M. Secondary myelofibrosis in visceral leishmaniasis--case report. Haematologia (Budap). 2001;31:167-71.

[44] Aggarwal P, Handa R, Singh S, Wali JP. Kala-azar--new developments in diagnosis and treatment. *Indian J Pediatr* 1999;66:63-71.

[45] Seimenis A, Morelli D, Mantovani A. Zoonoses in the Mediterranean region. *Ann Ist Super Sanita*. 2006;42(4):437-45.

[46] Oster CN, Tramont EC. Fever in a recent visitor to the Middle East. *Curr Clin Top Infect Dis*. 1993;13:57-73.

[47] Baker MS, Strunk HK. Medical aspects of Persian Gulf operations: serious infectious and communicable diseases of the Persian Gulf and Saudi Arabian Peninsula. *Mil Med*. 1991 Aug;156(8):385-90.

[48] Oldfield EC 3rd, Wallace MR, Hyams KC, Yousif AA, Lewis DE, Bourgeois AL. Endemic infectious diseases of the Middle East. *Rev Infect Dis*. 1991 Jan-Feb;13 Suppl 3:S199-217.

[49] Faulde M, Schrader J, Heyl G, Amirih M, Hoerauf A. Zoonotic cutaneous leishmaniasis outbreak in Mazar-e Sharif, northern Afghanistan: an epidemiological evaluation. *Int J Med Microbiol*. 2008 Jul;298(5-6):543-50.

[50] Leslie T, Saleheen S, Sami M, Mayan I, Mahboob N, Fiekert K, Lenglet A, Ord R, Reithinger R. Visceral leishmaniasis in Afghanistan. *CMAJ*. 2006 Aug 1;175(3):245.

[51] Nasereddin A, Baneth G, Schönian G, Kanaan M, Jaffe CL. Molecular fingerprinting of Leishmania infantum strains following an outbreak of visceral leishmaniasis in central Israel. *J Clin Microbiol*. 2005 Dec;43(12

[52] Yaghoobi-Ershadi MR, Jafari R, Hanafi-Bojd AA. A new epidemic focus of zoonotic cutaneous leishmaniasis in central Iran. *Ann Saudi Med*. 2004 Mar-Apr;24(2):98-101.

[53] Reithinger R, Aadil K, Hami S, Kolaczinski J. Cutaneous leishmaniasis, northern Afghanistan. *Emerg Infect Dis*. 2004 May;10(5):966-7.

[54] Reyburn H, Rowland M, Mohsen M, Khan B, Davies C. The prolonged epidemic of anthroponotic cutaneous leishmaniasis in Kabul, Afghanistan: 'bringing down the neighbourhood'. *Trans R Soc Trop Med Hyg*. 2003 Mar-Apr;97(2):170-6.

[55] Jacobson RL, Eisenberger CL, Svobodova M, Baneth G, Sztern J, Carvalho J, Nasereddin A, El Fari M, Shalom U, Volf P, Votypka J, Dedet JP, Pratlong F, Schonian G, Schnur LF, Jaffe CL, Warburg A. Outbreak of cutaneous leishmaniasis in northern northern Israel. *J Infect Dis*. 2003 Oct 1;188(7):1065-73. Epub 2003 Sep 22.

[56] Yaghoobi-Ershadi MR, Hanafi-Bojd AA, Javadian E, Jafari R, Zahraei-Ramazani AR, Mohebali M. A new focus of cutaneous leishmaniasis caused by Leishmania tropica. *Saudi Med J*. 2002 Mar;23(3):291-4.

[57] Volf P, Ozbel Y, Akkafa F, Svobodová M, Votýpka J, Chang KP. Sand flies (Diptera: Phlebotominae) in Sanliurfa, Turkey: relationship of Phlebotomus sergenti with the epidemic of anthroponotic cutaneous leishmaniasis. *J Med Entomol*. 2002 Jan;39(1):12-5.

[58] Yaghoobi-Ershadi MR, Hanafi-Bojd AA, Akhavan AA, Zahrai-Ramazani AR, Mohebali M. Epidemiological study in a new focus of cutaneous leishmaniosis due to Leishmania major in Ardestan town, central Iran. *Acta Trop*. 2001 May 25;79(2):115-21.

[59] Khoury S, Saliba EK, Oumeish OY. Short report: outbreak of cutaneous leishmaniasis in a nonimmune population of soldiers in Wadi Araba, Jordan.

[60] *Am J Trop Med Hyg*. 1999 Apr;60(4):520.

[61] Alptekin D, Kasap M, Luleyap U, Kasap H, Aksoy S, Wilson ML. Sandflies (Diptera: Psychodidae) associated with epidemic cutaneous leishmaniasis in Sanliurfa, Turkey. *J Med Entomol.* 1999 May;36(3):277-81.

[62] Tayeh A, Jalouk L, Cairncross S. Twenty years of cutaneous leishmaniasis in Aleppo, Syria. *Trans R Soc Trop Med Hyg.* 1997 Nov-Dec;91(6):657-9.

[63] Jumaian N, Kamhawi SA, Halalsheh M, Abdel-Hafez SK. Short report: outbreak of cutaneous leishmaniasis in a nonimmune population of soldiers in Wadi Araba, Jordan. *Am J Trop Med Hyg.* 1998 Feb;58(2):160-2.

[64] Gramiccia M, Bettini S, Yasarol S. Isoenzyme characterization of Leishmania isolates from human cases of cutaneous leishmaniasis in Urfa, south-east Turkey. *Trans R Soc Trop Med Hyg.* 1984;78(4):568.

[65] Büttiker W, Lewis DJ. Ecological studies at Hofuf, Eastern Saudi Arabia, in relation to dermal leishmaniasis. *Tropenmed Parasitol.* 1979 Jun;30(2):220-9.

[66] Nadim A, Seyedi-Rashti MA, Ashi J. Cutaneous leishmaniasis in Saudi-Arabia: an overview. *Bull Soc Pathol Exot Filiales.* 1979 May-Jun;72(3):237-44.

[67] Koufman Z, Egoz N. Nebi Mussa: a new focus of cutaneous leishmaniasis. *Harefuah.* 1978 Jul 2;95(1):8-9.

Chapter V

Dengue Virus Infection in India

Introduction to Dengue Fever

Dengue infection is a mosquito-borne arboviral infectious disease. The infection of the virus brings a variable spectrum of the illness that runs from a simple fever to severe dengue hemorrhagic fever (HDF), a fatal disease [1]. Mairuhu et al said that dengue fever came to be more recognized as one of the greater contagious illnesses owing to increased incident and spreading geographical distribution of dengue fever in the past years [1]. Nogueira said that dengue fever was one of the very frequent predominant acute fevers and might be extremely fatal if associated with complications [2]. Halstead said that the antibodies played significant roles in protecting and expanding infections of dengue fever, therefore, there are ongoing studies trying to find the final knowledge of what parts in the human body are infected by the human dengue fever and trying to gain a comprehension of early antibody-accessible steps of the infection concentrating on cellular level [3]. Nogueira also noted that control of vector was still the most effective means of preventive medicine [2]. There have been many efforts in the last six decades to produce a vaccine to fight this infection [4]. According to globalization in the present, the dengue fever shows arising patterns not only tropical but also in non-tropical countries. Wilson recently said that travelers could also be seen as carriers that harbor pathogen and microbial genetic matter to other regions of the world where investigators could carry out detailed analyses that could help map the location and movement of strains, genotypes and resistance patterns [5]. The knowledge about dengue infection is, therefore, an interesting theme for general physicians around the world.

Dengue in India

Dengue infection is an important vector-borne disease. With an annual incidence of millions of clinically diagnosed cases, dengue infection is still one of the top communicable diseases in the world. This reflects a need for intensive leishmanial control because dengue still continues to hit large populations in all parts of the tropics. Asia is an area stricken by the disease known as dengue. The endemic areas of dengue cover some specific areas of the Asian region. South Asia is one specific area experiencing a problem with dengue. In this chapter, the author uses the specific term of Indian dengue to describe the problem of dengue in South Asia.

Table 1. Reports on the emergence of dengue in India.

Author	Details
Kukreti et al [6]	Kukreti et al reported on emergence of an independent lineage of dengue virus type 1 (DENV-1) and its co-circulation with predominant DENV-3 during the 2006 dengue fever outbreak in Delhi, India [6].
Dash et al [7]	Dash et al reported on emergence of dengue virus type-3 in northern India [7].
Lal et al [8]	Lal et al reported on an emerging dengue fever in Ludhiana, North India [8].
Chandralekha et al [9]	Chandralekha et al reported on the north Indian dengue outbreak 2006 by a retrospective analysis of intensive care unit admissions in a tertiary care hospital [9].
Batra et al [10]	Batra et al reported on an outbreak of dengue infection in rural Maharashtra, India [10].
Samuel et al [11]	Samuel et al reported on a focal outbreak of dengue fever in a rural area of Tamil Nadu, India [11].
Balakrishnan et al [12]	Balakrishnan et al reported on an entomological study on the dengue vectors during outbreak of dengue in Tiruppur town and its surroundings, Tamil Nadu, India [12].
Paramasivan et al [13]	Paramasivan et al reported on a study on seroepidemiology of a focal outbreak of dengue in Tamil Nadu, India [13].
Kamal et al [14]	Kamal et al reported on an outbreak of dengue fever in Veerannapet village, Cherial Mandal, of Warangal district, Andhra Pradesh, India [14].
Paramasivan et al [15]	Paramasivan et al reported on serological and entomological investigations of an outbreak of dengue fever in certain rural areas of Kanyakumari district, Tamil Nadu, India [15].
Sharma et al [16]	Sharma et al reported on an outbreak of dengue in national capital territory of Delhi, India during 2003 [16]
Chakravarti and Kumaria [17]	Chakravarti and Kumaria reported on circulating levels of tumour necrosis factor-alpha and interferon-gamma in patients with dengue and dengue haemorrhagic fever during an outbreak in India [17].
Singh et al [18]	Singh et al reported on the 2003 outbreak of Dengue fever in Delhi, India [18].
Podder et al [19]	Podder et al noted that origin of dengue type 3 viruses in India associated with the dengue outbreak in Dhaka, Bangladesh, in 2000 and 2001 [19].

Ratho et al [20]	Ratho et al reported on an outbreak of dengue fever in periurban slums of Chandigarh, India, with special reference to entomological and climatic factors [20].
Dash et al [21]	Dash et al reported on an emergence of dengue virus type-3 in northern India [21].
Karande et al [22]	Karande et al reported on a concurrent outbreak of leptospirosis and dengue in Mumbai, India [22].
Chakravarti and Kumaria [23]	Chakravarti and Kumaria peformed an eco-epidemiological analysis of dengue infection during an outbreak of dengue fever, India [23].
Dutta et al [24]	Dutta et al reported on an entomological observation on dengue vector mosquitoes following a suspected outbreak of dengue in certain parts of Nagaland with a note on their susceptibility to insecticides [24].
Arya et al [25]	Arya et al reported on private sector hospital response to the 2003 dengue outbreak in the Indian capital metropolis of Delhi, India [25].
Shah et al [26]	Shah et al reported on an outbreak of dengue in Mumbai, India, and predictive markers for dengue shock syndrome [26].
Kabilan et al [27]	Kabilan et al reported on field- and laboratory-based active dengue surveillance in Chennai, Tamil Nadu, India focusing on the observations before and during the 2001 dengue epidemic [27].
Arunachalam et al [28]	Arunachalam et al reported on the studies on dengue in rural areas of Kurnool District, Andhra Pradesh, India [28].
Dash et al [29]	Dash et al reported on the emergence and continued circulation of dengue-2 (genotype IV) virus strains in northern India [29].
Kabilan et al [30]	Kabilan et al reported on dengue disease spectrum among infants in the 2001 dengue epidemic in Chennai, Tamil Nadu, India [30].
Parida et al [31]	Parida et al reported on serological and virological investigation of an outbreak of dengue fever in Gwalior, India [31].
Victor et al [32]	Victor et al reported on dengue fever outbreaks in two villages of Dharmapuri district in Tamil Nadu, India [32].
Kumar et al [33]	Kumar et al reported on platelet transfusion practice during dengue fever epidemic in India [33].
Kumar et al [34]	Kumar et al reported on an outbreak of dengue fever in rural areas of northern India [34].
Gokhale et al [35]	Gokhale et al reporeted on dengue virus and insecticide susceptibility status of *Aedes aegypti* mosquitoes from Belagola village, Mandya District, Karnataka state, India, during and post-epidemic investigations [35].
Tripathi et al [36]	Tripathi et al reported their experience in adult population in dengue outbreak in Delhi, India [36].

Joshi et al [37]	Joshi et al reported on and epidemiological and entomological investigation in dengue outbreak area of Ahmedabad district, India [37].
Singh et al ;38]	Singh et al reported on a silent spread of dengue and dengue haemorrhagic fever to Coimbatore and Erode districts in Tamil Nadu, India in 1998 [38].
Goel [39]	Goel reported on the dengue fever epidemic in Delhi, India [39].
Kabra et al [40]	Kabra et al reported on Dengue haemorrhagic fever in children in the 1996 Delhi epidemic [40].
Agarwal et al [41]	Agarwal et al reported a clinical study of the patients with dengue hemorrhagic fever during the epidemic of 1996 at Lucknow, India [41].
Dar et al [42]	Dar et al reported the first major outbreak of dengue hemorrhagic fever in Delhi, India [42].
Kabra et al [43]	Kabra et al reported on Dengue haemorrhagic fever in children in the 1996 Delhi epidemic [43].
Teichmann et al [44]	Teichmann et al reported on imported dengue virus type 2 infection acquired during an outbreak in India [44].
Aggarwal et al [45]	Aggarwal et al reported on an epidemic of dengue hemorrhagic fever and dengue shock syndrome in children in Delhi, India [45].
Kaul et al [46]	Kaul et al reported on preventing dengue and dengue haemorrhagic fever outbreaks in the National Capital Territory of Delhi based on entomological surveillance [46].
Gupta et al [47]	Gupta et al studied knowledge, attitude and practices related to dengue in rural and slum areas of Delhi after the dengue epidemic of 1996 [47].
Vaughn [48]	Vaughn performed a serological investigation of a febrile outbreak in Delhi, India, using a rapid immunochromatographic test [48].
Saxena et al [49]	Saxena et al described hemostatic abnormalities in dengue haemorrhagic fever in the New Delhi outbreak, India [49].
Kaur et al [50]	Kaur et al reported on dengue haemorrhagic fever outbreak in October-November 1996 in Ludhiana, Punjab, India [50].
Jamaluddain and Saxena [51]	Jamaluddain and Saxena reported on the first outbreak of Dengue fever in a typical rural area of Haryana state in northern India [51].
Abdul Kader et al [52]	Abdul Kader et al described outbreak and control of dengue in a village in Dharmapuri, Tamil Nadu, India [52].
Padbidri et al [53]	Padbidri et al reported on the 1993 epidemic of dengue fever in Mangalore, Karnataka state, India [53].
Cherian et al [54]	Cherian et al reported on an epidemic of dengue haemorrhagic fever and dengue shock syndrome in and around Vellore, India [54].
Bhattacharjee et al [55]	Bhattacharjee et al reported on dengue haemorrhagic fever outbreak in Calcutta in 1990 [55].

Mehendale et al [56]	Mehendale et al reported on an outbreak of dengue fever in rural areas of Parbhani district of Maharashtra, India [56].
Ilkal et al [57]	Ilkal et al reported on entomological investigations during outbreaks of dengue fever in certain villages in Maharashtra state, India [57].
Norman et al [58]	Norman et al reported on an insular outbreak of dengue fever in a rural south Indian village [58].
Chouhan et al [59]	Chouhan et al reported on clinical and virological study of dengue fever outbreak in Jalore city, Rajasthan, India [59].
Srivastava et al [60]	Srivastava et al reported a clinical study on an epidemic of dengue haemorrhagic fever and dengue shock syndrome in Delhi [60].
Acharya et al [61]	Acharya et al reported on an outbreak of Dengue fever in Delhi, India [61].
Chaturvedi et al [62]	Chaturvedi et al reported on a clinico-virological study of the recurrence of dengue epidemic with haemorrhagic manifestations at Kanpur during 1969 [62].
Myers et al [63]	Myers et al reported on the 1968 outbreak of dengue in Vellore, Southern India [63].
Myers et al [64]	Myers et al reported on dengue outbreak in Vellore, southern India, in 1968, with isolation of four dengue types from man and mosquitoes [64].
Myers et al [65]	Myers et al reported on dengue outbreak in Vellore, southern India, in 1968, with isolation of four dengue types from man and mosquitoes [65].
Chaturvedi et al [66]	Chaturvedi et al reported on a clinical and epidemiological study of an epidemic of febrile illness with haemorrhagic manifestations which occurred at Kanpur, India [66].
Chaturvedi et al [67]	Chaturvedi et al reported a virological study of an epidemic of febrile illness with haemorrhagic manifestations at Kanpur, India, during 1968 [67].
Myers et al [68]	Myers et al reported on virological investigations of the 1966 outbreak of Dengue type 3 in Vellore, Southern India [68].
Balaya et al [69]	Balaya et al reported investigations on an outbreak of dengue in Delhi in 1967 [69].
Chatterjee et al [70]	Chatterjee et al reported a virological investigation of cases with neurological complications during the outbreak of haemorrhagic fever in Calcutta, India [70].
Paul et al [71]	Paul et al reported on virological and serological studies on an outbreak of dengue-like illness in Visakhapatnam, Andhra Pradesh, India [71].
Krishnamurthy et al [72]	Krishnamurthy et al reported on clinical and pathological studies of an outbreak of dengue-like illness in Visakhapatnam, India [72].

1. Dengue in India

India is a big country. There are also some areas that lie in the tropical region. Therefore, the problem of dengue can be seen. The dengue can be classified as an important emerging infection in India. There are many reports on the emergence of dengue in India as shown in Table 1.

2. Dengue in Nepal

Nepal is another country in South Asia. There are no reports on the emergence of dengue in Nepal. This might be due to the fact that Nepal is not in the tropical area of Asia.

3. Dengue in Bhutan

Bhutan is another country in South Asia. There are no reports on the emergence of dengue in Bhutan. This might be due to the fact that Bhutan is not in the tropical area of Asia.

4. Dengue in Maldives

Maldives is another country in South Asia. Of interest, there are no reports on the emergence of dengue in Maldives although this country lies in tropical zone. This may be due to the fact that this country is a combination of several islands in the Indian ocean.

5. Dengue in Sri Lanka

Sri Lanka is another country in South Asia. There are some interesting reports on the outbreaks or epidemics of dengue in Sri Lanka (Table 2).

Table 2. Reports on the emergence of dengue in Sri Lanka.

Author	Details
Kularatne et al [73]	Kularatne et al reported on cardiac complications of a dengue fever outbreak in Sri Lanka, 2005 [73].
Malavige et al [74]	Malavige et al reported on patterns of disease in Sri Lankan dengue patients [74].
de Silva et al [75]	de Silva et al reported on serologic evidence for an epizootic dengue virus infecting toque macaques at Polonnaruwa, Sri Lanka [75].
Mendis et al [76]	Mendis et al reported on epidemiology of dengue-like fever in Sri Lanka [76].

6. Dengue in Bangladesh

Bangladesh is another country in South Asia. There are some interesting reports on the outbreaks or epidemics of dengue in Bangladesh. (Table 3).

Table 3. Reports on the emergence of dengue in Bangladesh..

Author	Details
Podder et al [19]	Podder et al noted that origin of dengue type 3 viruses in India was related to the dengue outbreak in Dhaka, Bangladesh [19].
Rahman et al [77]	Rahman et al reported on the first outbreak of dengue hemorrhagic fever, Bangladesh [77].
Aziz et al [78]	Aziz et al mentioned for predominance of the DEN-3 genotype during the recent dengue outbreak in Bangladesh [78].
Hossain et al [79]	Hossain et al mentioned for serologic evidence of dengue infection before onset of epidemic, Bangladesh [79].
Ali et al [80]	Ali et al reported on use of a geographic information system for defining spatial risk for dengue transmission in Bangladesh and mentioned for role for *Aedes albopictus* in an urban outbreak [80].
Wagatsuma et al [81]	Wagatsuma et al reported on dengue fever outbreak in a recreation club, Dhaka, Bangladesh [81].
LaRocque et al [82]	LaRocque et al reported on interesting observations on leptospirosis during dengue outbreak, Bangladesh [82].
Islam et al [83]	Islam et al reported on molecular characterization and clinical evaluation of dengue outbreak in 2002 in Bangladesh [83].
Rahim and Sikder [84]	Rahim and Sikder reported on clinicopathologic manifestations and outcome of dengue fever and dengue haemorrhagic fever in Bangladesh [84].

7. Dengue in Pakistan

Pakistan is another country in South Asia. There are some interesting reports on the outbreaks or epidemics of dengue in Pakistan (Table 4).

Table 4. Reports on the emergence of dengue in Pakistan.

Author	Details
Chan et al [85]	Chan et al reported on dengue haemorrhagic fever outbreak in Karachi, Pakistan, 1994 [85].
Ahmed et al [86]	Ahmed et al reported on Dengue fever outbreak in Karachi 2006 and studied the profile and outcome of children under 15 years of age in this specific outbreak [86].
Ahmed et al [87]	Ahmed et al reported on dengue fever outbreak with a clinical management experience [87].
Khan et al [88]	Khan et al reported on dengue outbreak in Karachi, Pakistan, 2006 showing experience at a tertiary care center [88].
Paul et al [89]	Paul et al reported on expansion of epidemic dengue viral infections to Pakistan [89].
Qureshi et al [90]	Qureshi et al reported on an epidemic of dengue fever in Karachi focusing on associated clinical manifestations [90].

References

[1] Mairuhu AT, Wagenaar J, Brandjes DP, van Gorp EC. Dengue: an arthropod-borne disease of global importance. *Eur J Clin Microbiol Infect Dis*. 2004; 23: 425-33.

[2] Nogueira SA. Dengue. *J Pediatr* (Rio J). 1999; 75(Suppl 1): S9-S14.

[3] Halstead SB. Dengue. *Curr. Opin Infect Dis*. 2002; 15: 471-6.

[4] Jacobs M, Young P. Dengue vaccines: preparing to roll back dengue. *Curr Opin Investig Drugs*. 2003; 4: 168-71.

[5] Wilson ME. The traveller and emerging infections: sentinel, courier, transmitter. *J Appl Microbiol*. 2003; 94 Suppl:1S-11S.

[6] Kukreti H, Chaudhary A, Rautela RS, Anand R, Mittal V, Chhabra M, Bhattacharya D, Lal S, Rai A. Emergence of an independent lineage of dengue virus type 1 (DENV-1) and its co-circulation with predominant DENV-3 during the 2006 dengue fever outbreak in Delhi. *Int J Infect Dis*. 2008 Sep;12(5):542-9.

[7] Dash PK, Saxena P, Abhyankar A, Bhargava R, Jana AM. Emergence of dengue virus type-3 in northern India. *Southeast Asian J Trop Med Public Health*. 2005 Mar;36(2):370-7.

[8] Lal M, Aggarwal A, Oberoi A. Dengue fever--an emerging viral fever in Ludhiana, North India. *Indian J Public Health*. 2007 Jul-Sep;51(3):198-9.

[9] Chandralekha, Gupta P, Trikha A. The north Indian dengue outbreak 2006: a retrospective analysis of intensive care unit admissions in a tertiary care hospital. *Trans R Soc Trop Med Hyg*. 2008 Feb;102(2):143-7.

[10] Batra P, Saha A, Chaturvedi P, Vilhekar KY, Mendiratta DK. Outbreak of dengue infection in rural Maharashtra. Indian J Pediatr. 2007 Aug;74(8):794-5

[11] Samuel PP, Thenmozhi V, Tyagi BK. A focal outbreak of dengue fever in a rural area of Tamil Nadu. *Indian J Med Res*. 2007 Feb;125(2):179-81

[12] Balakrishnan N, Venkatesh S, Lal S. An entomological study on the dengue vectors during outbreak of dengue in Tiruppur town and its surroundings, Tamil Nadu, India. *J Commun Dis.* 2006 Mar;38(2):164-8.

[13] Paramasivan R, Thenmozhi V, Kabilan L, Tewari SC, Arunachalam N, Dhananjeyan KJ, Tyagi BK. Seroepidemiology of a focal outbreak of dengue in Tamil Nadu. *Indian J Med Res.* 2006 Dec;124(6):718-20.

[14] Kamal S, Jain SK, Patnaik SK, Lal S. An outbreak of dengue fever in Veerannapet village, Cherial Mandal, of Warangal district, Andhra Pradesh. *J Commun Dis.* 2005 Dec;37(4):301-6.

[15] Paramasivan R, Thenmozhi V, Hiriyan J, Dhananjeyan K, Tyagi B, Dash AP. Serological and entomological investigations of an outbreak of dengue fever in certain rural areas of Kanyakumari district, Tamil Nadu. *Indian J Med Res.* 2006 May;123(5):697-701.

[16] Sharma RS, Joshi PL, Tiwari KN, Katyal R, Gill KS. Outbreak of dengue in national capital territory of Delhi, India during 2003. *J Vector Ecol.* 2005 Dec;30(2):337-8

[17] Chakravarti A, Kumaria R. Circulating levels of tumour necrosis factor-alpha & interferon-gamma in patients with dengue & dengue haemorrhagic fever during an outbreak. *Indian J Med Res.* 2006 Jan;123(1):25-30.

[18] Singh NP, Jhamb R, Agarwal SK, Gaiha M, Dewan R, Daga MK, Chakravarti A, Kumar S. The 2003 outbreak of Dengue fever in Delhi, India. *Southeast Asian J Trop Med Public Health.* 2005 Sep;36(5):1174-8.

[19] Podder G, Breiman RF, Azim T, Thu HM, Velathanthiri N, Mai le Q, Lowry K, Aaskov JG. Origin of dengue type 3 viruses associated with the dengue outbreak in Dhaka, Bangladesh, in 2000 and 2001. *Am J Trop Med Hyg.* 2006 Feb;74(2):263-5.

[20] Ratho RK, Mishra B, Kaur J, Kakkar N, Sharma K. An outbreak of dengue fever in periurban slums of Chandigarh, India, with special reference to entomological and climatic factors. *Indian J Med Sci.* 2005 Dec;59(12):518-26.

[21] Dash PK, Saxena P, Abhyankar A, Bhargava R, Jana AM. Emergence of dengue virus type-3 in northern India. *Southeast Asian J Trop Med Public Health.* 2005 Mar;36(2):370-7.

[22] Karande S, Gandhi D, Kulkarni M, Bharadwaj R, Pol S, Thakare J, De A. Concurrent outbreak of leptospirosis and dengue in Mumbai, India, 2002. *J Trop Pediatr.* 2005 Jun;51(3):174-81.

[23] Chakravarti A, Kumaria R. Eco-epidemiological analysis of dengue infection during an outbreak of dengue fever, India. *Virol J.* 2005 Apr 14;2:32.

[24] Dutta P, Khan SA, Khan AM, Sharma CK, Mahanta J. Entomological observations on dengue vector mosquitoes following a suspected outbreak of dengue in certain parts of Nagaland with a note on their susceptibility to insecticides. *J Environ Biol.* 2004 Apr;25(2):209-12.

[25] Arya SC, Rajagopal S, Agarwal N, Kaushik M, Maheshwari P, Agarwal S, Singh K, George S. Private sector hospital response to the 2003 dengue outbreak in the Indian capital metropolis of Delhi. *Am J Infect Control.* 2004 Dec;32(8):489-92.

[26] Shah I, Deshpande GC, Tardeja PN. Outbreak of dengue in Mumbai and predictive markers for dengue shock syndrome. *J Trop Pediatr.* 2004 Oct;50(5):301-5.

[27] Kabilan L, Velayutham T, Sundaram B, Tewari SC, Natarajan A, Rathnasamy R, Satyanarayana K. Field- and laboratory-based active dengue surveillance in Chennai, Tamil Nadu, India: observations before and during the 2001 dengue epidemic. *Am J Infect Control.* 2004 Nov;32(7):391-6.

[28] Arunachalam N, Murty US, Kabilan L, Balasubramanian A, Thenmozhi V, Narahari D, Ravi A, Satyanarayana K. Studies on dengue in rural areas of Kurnool District, Andhra Pradesh, India. *J Am Mosq Control Assoc.* 2004 Mar;20(1):87-90.

[29] Dash PK, Parida MM, Saxena P, Kumar M, Rai A, Pasha ST, Jana AM. Emergence and continued circulation of dengue-2 (genotype IV) virus strains in northern India. *J Med Virol.* 2004 Oct;74(2):314-22.

[30] Kabilan L, Balasubramanian S, Keshava SM, Thenmozhi V, Sekar G, Tewari SC, Arunachalam N, Rajendran R, Satyanarayana K. Dengue disease spectrum among infants in the 2001 dengue epidemic in Chennai, Tamil Nadu, India. *J Clin Microbiol.* 2003 Aug;41(8):3919-21.

[31] Parida MM, Dash PK, Upadhyay C, Saxena P, Jana AM. Serological & virological investigation of an outbreak of dengue fever in Gwalior, India. *Indian J Med Res.* 2002 Dec;116:248-54.

[32] Victor TJ, Malathi M, Gurusamy D, Desai A, Ravi V, Narayanasamy G, Anuradha L, Rani C, Krishnamurthy P. Dengue fever outbreaks in two villages of Dharmapuri district in Tamil Nadu. *Indian J Med Res.* 2002 Oct;116:133-9.

[33] Kumar ND, Tomar V, Singh B, Kela K. Platelet transfusion practice during dengue fever epidemic. *Indian J Pathol Microbiol.* 2000 Jan;43(1):55-60.

[34] Kumar A, Sharma SK, Padbidri VS, Thakare JP, Jain DC, Datta KK. An outbreak of dengue fever in rural areas of northern India. *J Commun Dis.* 2001 Dec;33(4):274-81.

[35] Gokhale MD, Jacob PG, Mourya DT. Dengue virus and insecticide susceptibility status of Aedes aegypti mosquitoes from Belagola village, Mandya District, Karnataka state: during and post-epidemic investigations. *J Commun Dis.* 2000 Dec;32(4):247-53.

[36] Tripathi BK, Gupta B, Sinha RS, Prasad S, Sharma DK. Experience in adult population in dengue outbreak in Delhi. *J Assoc Physicians India.* 1998 Mar;46(3):273-6.

[37] Joshi PT, Pandya AP, Anjan JK. Epidemiological and entomological investigation in dengue outbreak area of Ahmedabad district. *J Commun Dis.* 2000 Mar;32(1):22-7.

[38] Singh J, Balakrishnan N, Bhardwaj M, Amuthadevi P, George EG, Subramani K, Soundararajan K, Appavoo NC, Jain DC, Ichhpujani RL, Bhatia R, Sokhey J. Silent spread of dengue and dengue haemorrhagic fever to Coimbatore and Erode districts in Tamil Nadu, India, 1998: need for effective surveillance to monitor and control the disease. *Epidemiol Infect.* 2000 Aug;125(1):195-200.

[39] Goel A. The dengue fever epidemic in Delhi. J Assoc Physicians India. 1999 Jun;47(6):653-4.

[40] Kabra SK, Jain Y, Pandey RM, Madhulika, Singhal T, Tripathi P, Broor S, Seth P, Seth V. Dengue haemorrhagic fever in children in the 1996 Delhi epidemic. Trans R Soc Trop Med Hyg. 1999 May-Jun;93(3):294-8.

[41] Agarwal R, Kapoor S, Nagar R, Misra A, Tandon R, Mathur A, Misra AK, Srivastava KL, Chaturvedi UC. A clinical study of the patients with dengue hemorrhagic fever

during the epidemic of 1996 at Lucknow, India. *Southeast Asian J Trop Med Public* Health. 1999 Dec;30(4):735-40.

[42] Dar L, Broor S, Sengupta S, Xess I, Seth P. The first major outbreak of dengue hemorrhagic fever in Delhi, India. *Emerg Infect Dis*. 1999 Jul-Aug;5(4):589-90.

[43] Kabra SK, Jain Y, Pandey RM, Madhulika, Singhal T, Tripathi P, Broor S, Seth P, Seth V. Dengue haemorrhagic fever in children in the 1996 Delhi epidemic. Trans R Soc *Trop Med Hyg*. 1999 May-Jun;93(3):294-8.

[44] Teichmann D, Rögler G, Grobusch MP, Schüler-Maué W, Klein E. Imported dengue virus type 2 infection acquired during an outbreak in India. *Eur J Clin Microbiol Infect* Dis. 1999 Apr;18(4):310-2

[45] Aggarwal A, Chandra J, Aneja S, Patwari AK, Dutta AK. An epidemic of dengue hemorrhagic fever and dengue shock syndrome in children in Delhi. *Indian Pediatr*. 1998 Aug;35(8):727-32.

[46] Kaul SM, Sharma RS, Sharma SN, Panigrahi N, Phukan PK, Lal S. Preventing dengue/dengue haemorrhagic fever outbreaks in the National Capital Territory of Delhi--the role of entomological surveillance. *J Commun Dis*. 1998 Sep;30(3):187-92.

[47] Gupta P, Kumar P, Aggarwal OP.Knowledge, attitude and practices related to dengue in rural and slum areas of Delhi after the dengue epidemic of 1996. *J Commun Dis*. 1998 Jun;30(2):107-12.

[48] Vaughn DW. Serological investigation of a febrile outbreak in Delhi, India, using a rapid immunochromatographic test. *J Clin Microbiol*. 1998 Sep;36(9):2795-6.

[49] Saxena R, Bhargava M, Wali JP, Mishra DK, Mohanty S. Haemostatic abnormalities in dengue haemorrhagic fever in the New Delhi outbreak, India. *Am J Hematol*. 1998 Feb;57(2):183-4.

[50] Kaur H, Prabhakar H, Mathew P, Marshalla R, Arya M. Dengue haemorrhagic fever outbreak in October-November 1996 in Ludhiana, Punjab, India. *Indian J Med Res*. 1997 Jul;106:1-3.

[51] Jamaluddain M, Saxena VK. First outbreak of Dengue fever in a typical rural area of Haryana state in northern India. *J Commun Dis*. 1997 Jun;29(2):169-70

[52] Abdul Kader MS, Kandaswamy P, Appavoo NC, Anuradha. Outbreak and control of dengue in a village in Dharmapuri, Tamil Nadu. *J Commun Dis*. 1997 Mar;29(1):69-71

[53] Padbidri VS, Adhikari P, Thakare JP, Ilkal MA, Joshi GD, Pereira P, Guttikar SN, Walhekar BD, Chowta N, Hegde BM. The 1993 epidemic of dengue fever in Mangalore, Karnataka state, India. *Southeast Asian J Trop Med Public Health*. 1995 Dec;26(4):699-704.

[54] Cherian T, Ponnuraj E, Kuruvilla T, Kirubakaran C, John TJ, Raghupathy P. An epidemic of dengue haemorrhagic fever & dengue shock syndrome in & around Vellore. *Indian J Med Res*. 1994 Aug;100:51-6.

[55] Bhattacharjee N, Mukherjee KK, Chakravarti SK, Mukherjee MK, De PN, Sengupta M, Banik GB, Bhowmick P, Sinha SK, Chakraborty MS. Dengue haemorrhagic fever (DHF) outbreak in Calcutta--1990. *J Commun Dis*. 1993 Mar;25(1):10-4.

[56] Mehendale SM, Risbud AR, Rao JA, Banerjee K. Outbreak of dengue fever in rural areas of Parbhani district of Maharashtra (India). *Indian J Med Res*. 1991 Jan;93:6-11.

[57] Ilkal MA, Dhanda V, Hassan MM, Mavale M, Mahadev PV, Shetty PS, Guttikar SN, Banerjee K. Entomological investigations during outbreaks of dengue fever in certain villages in Maharashtra state. *Indian J Med Res.* 1991 May;93:174-8.

[58] Norman G, Theodre A, Joseph A. An insular outbreak of dengue fever in a rural south Indian village. *J Commun Dis.* 1991 Sep;23(3):185-90.

[59] Chouhan GS, Rodrigues FM, Shaikh BH, Ilkal MA, Khangaro SS, Mathur KN, Joshi KR, Vaidhye NK. Clinical & virological study of dengue fever outbreak in Jalore city, Rajasthan 1985. *Indian J Med Res.* 1990 Nov;91:414-8.

[60] Srivastava VK, Suri S, Bhasin A, Srivastava L, Bharadwaj M. An epidemic of dengue haemorrhagic fever and dengue shock syndrome in Delhi: a clinical study. *Ann Trop Paediatr.* 1990;10(4):329-34.

[61] Acharya SK, Buch P, Irshad M, Gandhi BM, Joshi YK, Tandon BN. Outbreak of Dengue fever in Delhi. *Lancet.* 1988 Dec 24-31;2(8626-8627):1485-6.

[62] Chaturvedi UC, Mathur A, Kapoor AK, Tandon HO, Mehrotra RM. Clinico-virological study of the recurrence of dengue epidemic with haemorrhagic manifestations at Kanpur during 1969. *Indian J Med Res.* 1972 Mar;60(3):329-33.

[63] Myers RM, Varkey MJ, Reuben R, Jesudass ES, Benjamin B. The 1968 outbreak of dengue in Vellore, Southern India. *Am J Public Health.* 1971 Jul;61(7):1379-91.

[64] Myers RM, Varkey MJ, Reuben R, Jesudass ES. Dengue outbreak in Vellore, southern India, in 1968, with isolation of four dengue types from man and mosquitoes. *Indian J Med Res.* 1970 Jan;58(1):24-30

[65] Myers RM, Varkey MJ, Reuben R, Jesudass ES. Dengue outbreak in Vellore, southern India, in 1968, with isolation of four dengue types from man and mosquitoes. *Indian J Med Res.* 1970 Jan;58(1):24-30.

[66] Chaturvedi UC, Kapoor AK, Mathur A, Chandra D, Khan AM, Mehrotra RM. A clinical and epidemiological study of an epidemic of febrile illness with haemorrhagic manifestations which occurred at Kanpur, India, in 1968. *Bull World Health Organ.* 1970;43(2):281-7. No

[67] Chaturvedi UC, Mathur A, Kapoor AK, Mehrotra NK, Mehrotra RM. Virological study of an epidemic of febrile illness with haemorrhagic manifestations at Kanpur, India, during 1968. *Bull World Health Organ.* 1970;43(2):289-93

[68] Myers RM, Carey DE, DeRanitz CM, Reuben R, Bennet B. Virological investigations of the 1966 outbreak of Dengue type 3 in Vellore, Southern India. *Indian J Med Res.* 1969 Aug;57(8):1392-401.

[69] Balaya S, Paul SD, D'Lima LV, Pavri KM. Investigations on an outbreak of dengue in Delhi in 1967. *Indian J Med Res.* 1969 Apr;57(4):767-74.

[70] Chatterjee SN, Chakravarti SK, Mitra AC, Sarkar JK. Virological investigation of cases with neurological complications during the outbreak of haemorrhagic fever in Calcutta. *J Indian Med Assoc.* 1965 Sep 16;45(6):314-6

[71] Paul SD, Dandawate CN, Banerjee K, Krishnamurthy K. Virological and serological studies on an outbreak of dengue-like illness in Visakhapatnam, Andhra Pradesh. *Indian J Med Res.* 1965 Aug;53(8):777-89.

[72] Krishnamurthy K, Kasturi TE, Chittipantulu G. Clinical and pathological studies of an outbreak of dengue-like illness in Visakhapatnam. *Indian J Med Res.* 1965 Aug;53(8):800-12.

[73] Kularatne SA, Pathirage MM, Kumarasiri PV, Gunasena S, Mahindawanse SI. Cardiac complications of a dengue fever outbreak in Sri Lanka, 2005. *Trans R Soc Trop Med Hyg.* 2007 Aug;101(8):804-8

[74] Malavige GN, Ranatunga PK, Velathanthiri VG, Fernando S, Karunatilaka DH, Aaskov J, Seneviratne SL. Patterns of disease in Sri Lankan dengue patients. *Arch Dis Child.* 2006 May;91(5):396-400.

[75] de Silva AM, Dittus WP, Amerasinghe PH, Amerasinghe FP. Serologic evidence for an epizootic dengue virus infecting toque macaques (Macaca sinica) at Polonnaruwa, Sri Lanka. *Am J Trop Med Hyg.* 1999 Feb;60(2):300-6.

[76] Mendis NM. Epidemiology of dengue-like fever in Ceylon. *Ceylon Med J.* 1967 Jun;12(2):67-74

[77] Rahman M, Rahman K, Siddque AK, Shoma S, Kamal AH, Ali KS, Nisaluk A, Breiman RF. First outbreak of dengue hemorrhagic fever, Bangladesh. *Emerg Infect Dis.* 2002 Jul;8(7):738-40.

[78] Aziz MM, Hasan KN, Hasanat MA, Siddiqui MA, Salimullah M, Chowdhury AK, Ahmed M, Alam MN, Hassan MS. Predominance of the DEN-3 genotype during the recent dengue outbreak in Bangladesh. *Southeast Asian J Trop Med Public Health.* 2002 Mar;33(1):42-8.

[79] Hossain MA, Khatun M, Arjumand F, Nisaluk A, Breiman RF. Serologic evidence of dengue infection before onset of epidemic, Bangladesh. *Emerg Infect Dis.* 2003 Nov;9(11):1411-4.

[80] Ali M, Wagatsuma Y, Emch M, Breiman RF. Use of a geographic information system for defining spatial risk for dengue transmission in Bangladesh: role for Aedes albopictus in an urban outbreak. *Am J Trop Med Hyg.* 2003 Dec;69(6):634-40.

[81] Wagatsuma Y, Breiman RF, Hossain A, Rahman M. Dengue fever outbreak in a recreation club, Dhaka, Bangladesh. *Emerg Infect Dis.* 2004 Apr;10(4):747-50.

[82] LaRocque RC, Breiman RF, Ari MD, Morey RE, Janan FA, Hayes JM, Hossain MA, Brooks WA, Levett PN. Leptospirosis during dengue outbreak, *Bangladesh. Emerg Infect Dis.* 2005 May;11(5):766-9.

[83] Islam MA, Ahmed MU, Begum N, Chowdhury NA, Khan AH, Parquet Mdel C, Bipolo S, Inoue S, Hasebe F, Suzuki Y, Morita K. Molecular characterization and clinical evaluation of dengue outbreak in 2002 in Bangladesh. Jpn J Infect Dis. 2006 Apr;59(2):85-91.

[84] Rahim MA, Sikder MS. Clinicopathologic manifestations and outcome of dengue fever and dengue haemorrhagic fever. *Bangladesh Med Res Counc Bull.* 2005 Apr;31(1):36-45.

[85] Chan YC, Salahuddin NI, Khan J, Tan HC, Seah CL, Li J, Chow VT. Dengue haemorrhagic fever outbreak in Karachi, Pakistan, 1994. *Trans R Soc Trop Med Hyg.* 1995 Nov-Dec;89(6):619-20.

[86] Ahmed S, Arif F, Yahya Y, Rehman A, Abbas K, Ashraf S, Akram DS. Dengue fever outbreak in Karachi 2006--a study of profile and outcome of children under 15 years of age. *J Pak Med Assoc*. 2008 Jan;58(1):4-8.

[87] Ahmed S, Ali N, Ashraf S, Ilyas M, Tariq WU, Chotani RA. Dengue fever outbreak: a clinical management experience. *J Coll Physicians Surg Pak*. 2008 Jan;18(1):8-12.

[88] Khan E, Siddiqui J, Shakoor S, Mehraj V, Jamil B, Hasan R. Dengue outbreak in Karachi, Pakistan, 2006: experience at a tertiary care center. *Trans R Soc Trop Med Hyg*. 2007 Nov;101(11):1114-9

[89] Paul RE, Patel AY, Mirza S, Fisher-Hoch SP, Luby SP. Expansion of epidemic dengue viral infections to Pakistan. *Int J Infect Dis*. 1998 Apr-Jun;2(4):197-201.

[90] Qureshi JA, Notta NJ, Salahuddin N, Zaman V, Khan JA. An epidemic of Dengue fever in Karachi--associated clinical manifestations. *J Pak Med Assoc*. 1997 Jul;47(7):178-81.

Chapter VI

Chikungunya Fever in India

Introduction to Chikungunya Fever

Chikungunya fever is a viral infection generating hemorrhagic fever similar to the dengue virus infection. Chikungunya virus is noted as an arbovirus in group A.

It is classified as a virus in the family Togaviridae [1]. Chikungunya fever is a viral disease transmitted to human beings by Aedes genus mosquitoes [1]. The chikungunya virus is highly infective and its incubation period is 3-12 days [2 - 3]. With regard to the clinical manifestations, sudden severe headache, the colds, fever, joint pain and myalgia are the most common symptoms [3]. Children can also show additional neurological symptoms [3]. The hemorrhagic fever is a serious complication of this infection; however, the hemorrhage is not common and can recede in 3-5 days [3]. Antigens or antibody study is the main diagnosis for this infection. An IgM ELISA is necessary to make differential diagnoses of dengue fever [3]. The application of the molecular diagnosis of the infection of Chikungunya virus has also been noted in medicine for the past few years [3]. The acute hemorrhagic fever of caused by Chikungunya infection can be managed with the similar protocols to dengue fever.

Chikungunya Fever in India

Chikungunya infection is an important vector-borne disease. With an annual incidence of millions of clinically diagnosed cases, Chikungunya infection is still one of the main arboviral infection of the world. This reflects a need for intensive leishmanial control because Chikungunya still continues to affect a lot of global populations in the tropical region of the world. Asia is an area of Chikungunya. The endemic areas of Chikungunya cover some specific areas of the Asian region. South Asia is the specifically mentioned area which confirms having the problem of Chikungunya . In this chapter, the author uses the specific term of Indian Chikungunya to describe the problem of Chikungunya in South Asia.

1. Chikungunya in India

India is a big country. There are also some areas that lie in the tropical region. Therefore, the problem of Chikungunya can be seen. Chikungunya can be classified as an important emerging infection in India. There are many reports on the emergence of Chikungunya in India as shown in Table 1.

Table 1. Reports on the emergence of Chikungunya in India.

Author	Details
Kumar et al [4]	Kumar et al reported on an A226V mutation in virus during the 2007 chikungunya outbreak in Kerala, India [4].
Kumar et al [5]	Kumar et al reported on an investigation of an outbreak of chikungunya in Malegaon Municipal areas of Nasik district, Maharashtra (India) and its control [5].
Inamadar et al [6]	Inamadar et al reported on cutaneous manifestations of chikungunya fever observed during a recent outbreak in south India [6].
Dash et al [7]	Dash et al mentioned that the Central South African genotype was the causative agent in reemergence of Chikungunya outbreak in India [7].
Manimunda et al [8]	Manimunda et al reported the emergence of Chikungunya fever in Andaman and Nicobar Islands, India [8].
Arankalle et al [9]	Arankalle et al mentioned genetic divergence of Chikungunya viruses in India (1963-2006) with special reference to the 2005-2006 explosive epidemic [9].
Padbidri and Ganeswar [10]	Padbidri and Ganeswar reported on epidemiological investigations of chikungunya epidemic at Barsi, Maharashtra state, India [10].
Carey et al [11]	Carey et al reported on the 1964 chikungunya epidemic at Vellore, South India, including observations on concurrent dengue [11].
Reuben [12]	Reuben mentioned some entomological and epidemiological observations on the 1964 outbreak of Chikungunya fever in South India [12].

2. Chikungunya in Nepal

Nepal is another country in South Asia. There are no reports on the emergence of Chikungunya in Nepal. This might be due to the fact that Nepal is not in the tropical area of Asia.

3. Chikungunya in Bhutan

Bhutan is another country in South Asia. There are no reports on the emergence of Chikungunya in Bhutan. This might be due to the fact that Bhutan is not in the tropical area of Asia.

4. Chikungunya in Maldives

Maldives is another country in South Asia. Of interest, there are no reports on the emergence of Chikungunya in Maldives although this country lies in tropical zone. This may be due to the fact that this country is a combination of several islands in the Indian ocean.

5. Chikungunya in Sri Lanka

Sri Lanka is another country in South Asia. There are some interesting reports on the outbreaks or epidemics of Chikungunya in Sri Lanka (Table 2).

Table 2. Reports on the emergence of Chikungunya in Sri Lanka.

Author	Details
Hermon [13]	Hermon performed virological investigations of Arbovirus infections in Sri Lanka, with special reference to the recent Chikungunya fever epidemic [13]

6. Chikungunya in Bangladesh

Bangladesh is another country in South Asia. However, there is no report on the emergence of Chikungunya in Bangladesh.

7. Chikungunya in Pakistan

Pakistan is another country in South Asia. However, there is no report on the emergence of Chikungunya in Pakistan.

Pathogenesis, Diagnosis and Treatment of Chikungunya Infection at Present

The pathogenesis of Chikungunya infection is the same process as that of dengue fever. Hemorrhagic episodes are believed to be immunological pathways. Arthritis seems to be due to this the same process. For the outbreak, the molecular shift is also significant. The unique molecular features of the analyzed Indian Ocean isolates of chikungunya virus shows their high evolutionary potential and suggest feasibility to understand the atypical magnitude and virulence of the recent outbreak in Indian Ocean territories [9, 14]. Clinical manifestation of Chikungunya virus infection is similar to that of dengue infection and is characterized by fever, eruptions and invalidating arthralgia [15 - 16]. Although viral diagnostics (culture, serological tests and polymerase chain reaction tests) can be applied to confirm the infection, these tests are not accessible during outbreaks to most of the population in the poor underdeveloped endemic areas [17]. Chikungunya fever should be a concern for travelers who develop fever and arthritis returning from the specific areas affected by an ongoing epidemic [18]. Related arthritis mainly hits smaller joints and often persists for extended periods [18]. Serological testing can also give negative results during the first week of the disease therefore diagnosis using polymerase chain reaction can bring more reliability during this time [18].

Similar to dengue infection, there is no specific treatment for Chikunganya infection, therefore, symptomatic treatment, especially for fluid replacement therapy is recommended. There is some ongoing clinical research on the use of chloroquine for treatment of chronic arthritis in Chikunganya infection [19]. About one-tenth of patients who contract Chikungunya virus infection develop chronic joint symptoms and the symptoms usually respond only partially to the non-steroidal anti-inflammatory drugs [19]. However, there is no clear evidence that chloroquine is effective for relieving or treatment of the described symptoms.

References

[1] Diallo M, Thonnon J, Traore-Lamizana M, Fontenille D. Vectors of Chikungunya virus in Senegal: current data and transmission cycles.*Am J Trop Med Hyg*. 1999; 60: 281-6.

[2] Chikungunya infection. Available at http://www.cbwinfo.com/Biological/Pathogens/CHIK.html

[3] Andrei G, De Clercq E. Molecular approaches for the treatment of hemorrhagic fever virus infections. *Antiviral Res*. 1993; 22: 45-75.

[4] Kumar NP, Joseph R, Kamaraj T, Jambulingam P. A226V mutation in virus during

[5] the 2007 chikungunya outbreak in Kerala, *India. J Gen Virol*. 2008 Aug;89(Pt 8):1945-8.

[6] Kumar K, Chhabra M, Katyal R, Patnaik PK, Kukreti H, Rai A, Saxena VK, Mittal V, Lal S. Investigation of an outbreak of chikungunya in Malegaon Municipal areas of

Nasik district, Maharashtra (India) and its control. *J Vector Borne Dis.* 2008 Jun;45(2):157-63.

[7] Inamadar AC, Palit A, Sampagavi VV, Raghunath S, Deshmukh NS. Cutaneous manifestations of chikungunya fever: observations made during a recent outbreak in south India. *Int J Dermatol.* 2008 Feb;47(2):154-9.

[8] Dash PK, Parida MM, Santhosh SR, Verma SK, Tripathi NK, Ambuj S, Saxena P, Gupta N, Chaudhary M, Babu JP, Lakshmi V, Mamidi N, Subhalaxmi MV, Lakshmana Rao PV, Sekhar K. East Central South African genotype as the causative agent in reemergence of Chikungunya outbreak in India. *Vector Borne Zoonotic Dis.* 2007 Winter;7(4):519-27.

[9] Manimunda SP, Singh SS, Sugunan AP, Singh O, Roy S, Shriram AN, Bharadwaj AP, Shah WA, Vijayachari P. Chikungunya fever, Andaman and Nicobar Islands, India. *Emerg Infect Dis.* 2007 Aug;13(8):1259-60.

[10] Arankalle VA, Shrivastava S, Cherian S, Gunjikar RS, Walimbe AM, Jadhav SM, Sudeep AB, Mishra AC. Genetic divergence of Chikungunya viruses in India (1963-2006) with special reference to the 2005-2006 explosive epidemic. *J Gen Virol.* 2007 Jul;88(Pt 7):1967-76.

[11] Padbidri VS, Gnaneswar TT. Epidemiological investigations of chikungunya epidemic at Barsi, Maharashtra state, India. *J Hyg Epidemiol Microbiol Immunol.* 1979; 23(4):445-51.

[12] Carcy DE, Myers RM, DeRanitz CM, Jadhav M, Reuben R. The 1964 chikungunya epidemic at Vellore, South India, including observations on concurrent dengue. *Trans R Soc Trop Med Hyg.* 1969;63(4):434-45.

[13] Reuben R. Some entomological and epidemiological observations on the 1964 outbreak of Chikungunya fever in South India. *Indian J Med Res.* 1967 Jan;55(1):1-12.

[14] Hermon YE. Virological investigations of Arbovirus infections in Ceylon, with special reference to the recent Chikungunya fever epidemic. *Ceylon Med J.* 1967 Jun;12(2):81-92.

[15] 14.Schuffenecker I, Iteman I, Michault A, Murri S, Frangeul L, Vaney MC, Lavenir R, Pardigon N, Reynes JM, Pettinelli F, Biscornet L, Diancourt L, Michel S, Duquerroy S, Guigon G, Frenkiel MP, Brehin AC, Cubito N, Despres P, Kunst F, Rey FA, Zeller H, Brisse S. Genome microevolution of chikungunya viruses causing the Indian Ocean outbreak. *PLoS Med.* 2006; 3: e263.

[16] 15.Nakoune E, Finance C, Le Faou A, Rihn B. The Chikungunya virus. *Ann Biol Clin* (Paris). 2007; 65: 349-56.

[17] 16.Mohan A. Chikungunya fever: clinical manifestations & management. Indian. *J. Med Res.* 2006; 124: 471-4 (2006)

[18] 17.Kalantri SP, Joshi R, Riley LW. Chikungunya epidemic: an Indian perspective. *Natl Med J India.* 2006; 19: 315-22.

[19] 18.Taubitz W, Cramer JP, Kapaun A, Pfeffer M, Drosten C, Dobler G, Burchard GD, Loscher T. Chikungunya fever in travelers: clinical presentation and course. *Clin Infect Dis.* 2007; 45: e1-4.

[20] 19. Brighton SW. Chloroquine phosphate treatment of chronic Chikungunya arthritis. An open pilot study. *S Afr Med J.* 1984; 66: 217-8..

Chapter VII

Japanese Encephalitis in India

Introduction to Japanese Encephalitis

Japanese encephalitis is another mosquito-borne arboviral infection [1]. Globally, the Japanese encephalitis virus is arising as a more important viral encephalitis despite the vaccine being available [2]. Solomon said that recent work on the Japanese encephalitis virus suggested that the virus has its origin in the specific area of Indonesian-Malaya, and in some extending areas [2]. For a few years, significant advances have been made due to the understanding of natural history and pathogenesis of this deadly mosquito borne viral encephalitis [3]. Mackenzie et al noted that mosquito-borne flaviviruses inclusive Japanese encephalitis virus provided some of the most important examples to arise on resurging infections of global significance [4]. Gubler said that there had been a resurgence or dramatic increase of illnesses of arboviral or epidemic including Japanese encephalitis, affecting both humans and pets [5]. Zeller said that the air transportation permitted the fast changing site from place to place as well as the diffusion of potential vectors and infected host [6].

Today this illness still affects many humans, especially in Asia, and places a significant danger to unvaccinated travelers to this region [7]. This illness can be classified as classical viral encephalitis and can be diagnosed using serology, by the isolation of virus, or by the molecular diagnosis technique [1]. The illness associates with a severe encephalitis, a high mortality and a high incident of neurological sequelae in the ones who can survive the infection [8].

Although there have been many efforts for decades to be rid of this illness the infection still exists in many settings. As a zoonosis, Japanese encephalitis cannot be eradicated, but the minimization of the human load of the illness is probable by routine vaccination of children in endemic countries; with a low cost compared to the expected benefits [1]. According to present globalization, the Japanese encephalitis arises as an infectious problem not only for tropical but also to for non-tropical countries. Vaccination for the traveler is recommended for Japanese encephalitis [7 - 9]. The knowledge on Japanese encephalitis is, therefore, an interesting and important topic for general doctors throughout the world.

How Can Japanese Encephalitis Become an Emerging Infectious Disease in a New Setting?

As already mentioned, Japanese encephalitis is classified as an important vector borne disease. Mosquitos are the main vector for this infection. It can be said that the mosquito is an insect that can fly and can spread the disease widely. Many important mosquito borne diseases emerged within the past few years due to many reasons. The first thing to be mentioned is the mosquito is usually prevalent in the tropical region. The change of the global climate due to global warming phenomenon can help spread the geoendemic size of problematic mosquitoes. This can bring the new emergence of many mosquito borne infectious diseases in the new settings. In addition, the mosquito vector of Japanese encephalitis is classified as an urban mosquito. This is different from the mosquito vector of malaria which is classified as a forest hospital. Therefore, the crowded population in the city, especially in crowded places, help generate contact to the vector mosquito. Poor sanitation in the crowded places is usually due to poverty. This has already been mentioned several times. Poor sanitation promotes the generalization of mosquito vectors and can result in the epidemic of Japanese encephalitis. How to mange the poverty seems to be the key for sanitation development and the consequent reduction of the rate of Japanese encephalitis infections. This can be helpful for the improvement of health status; not only for Japanese encephalitis but also for other health disorders.

Another point to be mentioned is the fact that the mosquito vector tends to develop resistance to insecticide. In the present day, insecticide is widely used in the city and this can be the root cause for the emergence of insecticide resistant mosquito vector. This can prevent the success in mosquito control. Finally, the direct rapid distribution of the mosquito vector to the new setting should be noted. This can be explained by the good transportation at present. The mosquito vector can be delivered from endemic area to new places via the airplane. This can be seen in some imported cases of mosquito borne infectious disease in new countries. This phenomenon existed in the literature. Conclusively, all described processes are not specific to Japanese encephalitis but can be applied for other emerging mosquito borne infectious diseases.

Japanese Encephalitis in India

Japanese encephalitis infection is an important vector-borne disease. With an annual incidence of millions of clinically diagnosed cases, Japanese encephalitis infection is still one of the main arboviral infections of the world. This reflects a need for Japanese encephalitis virus intensive control because Japanese encephalitis still continues to affect a lot of global populations in the tropical region of the world. Asia is an area experiencing problems with this virus. The endemic areas of Japanese encephalitis cover some specific areas of the Asian region. South Asia is the specifically mentioned area confirming having the problem of Japanese encephalitis. In this chapter, the author uses the specific term of Indian Japanese encephalitis to describe the problem of Japanese encephalitisin in South Asia.

Table 1. Reports on the emergence of Japanese encephalitis in India.

Author	Details
Kanojia and Jamgaonkar [10]	Kanojia and Jamgaonkar described a study focusing on mosquito records from a hot and dry climatic area experiencing frequent outbreaks of Japanese encephalitis, Bellary district, Karnataka, India [10].
Gupta et al [11]	Gupta et al reported on negligible case fatality due to Japanese encephalitis owing to an outbreak investigation in 2004 [11]
Parida et al [12]	Parida et al reported on Japanese Encephalitis Outbreak, India, 2005 [12].
Lawrence [13]	Lawrence reported on Japanese encephalitis outbreak in India and Nepal [13].
Kumar [14]	Kumar reported on clinical features in children hospitalized during the 2005 epidemic of Japanese encephalitis in Uttar Pradesh, India [14].
Gupta et al [15]	Gupta et al reported on epidemiological profile of Japanese encephalitis outbreak in Gorakhpur, UP in 2004 [15].
Rao et al [16]	Rao et al reported an outbreak of Japanese encephalitis in Haryana, India [16].
Mudur et al [17]	Mudur noted that Japanese encephalitis outbreak killed up to 1,300 children in India [17]
Chatterjee [18]	Chatterjee reported a Japanese encephalitis outbreak in India [18].
Raut et al [19]	Raut et al reported a focal outbreak of Japanese Encephalitis among horses in Pune district, India [19]
Kaur [20]	Kaur reported an investigation into the JE epidemic of 2000 in Upper Assam [20].
Arunachalam et al [21]	Arunachalam et al reported on vertical transmission of Japanese encephalitis virus in Mansonia species, in an epidemic-prone area of southern India [21]
Rao et al [22]	Rao et al reported on Japanese Encephalitis epidemic in Anantapur district, Andhra Pradesh, India during October-November, 1999 [22].
Dash et al [23]	Dash et al reported a retrospective analysis of epidemiological investigation of Japanese encephalitis outbreak occurred in Rourkela, Orissa, India [23].
CDC [24]	Outbreak news on Japanese encephalitis, India was reported [2.4]
Neogi et al [25]	Neogi et al reported on detection of HIV seropositivity during an outbreak of Japanese encephalitis in Manipur, India [25].
Dhanda et al [26]	Dhanda et al reported on virus isolation from wild-caught mosquitoes during a Japanese encephalitis outbreak in Kerala in 1996 [26].
Rathi et al [27]	Rathi et al reported on JE virus encephalitis outbreak in 1988 epidemic at Gorakhpur, India [27].
Vajpayee [28]	Vajpayee reported on a study of the outbreak of Japanese encephalitis in Lakhimpur district of Assam in 1989 [28].
Sharma and Panwar [29]	Sharma and Panwar reported on an epidemic of Japanese encephalitis in Haryana in the year 1990 [29].

Sharma et al [30]	Sharma et al reported on an outbreak of Japanese encephalitis in Haryana, India [30].
Vajpayee et al [31]	Vajpayee et al mentioned an investigation of an outbreak of Japanese encephalitis in Rourkela City (Orissa) during 1989 [31].
Mukherjee et al [32]	Mukherjee et al reported on recurrent outbreaks of Japanese encephalitis in Nagaland during 1985-1989 by a seroepidemiological study [32].
Narasimham et al [33]	Narasimham et al reported an epidemiological investigation on Japanese encephalitis outbreak in Uttar Pradesh during 1988 [33].
Chakraborty et al [34]	Chakraborty et al reported on an outbreak of Japanese encephalitis in two districts of Assam during 1980 focusing on some epidemiological features [34].
Rao et al [35]	Rao et al reported on the 1981 epidemic of Japanese encephalitis in Tamil Nadu and Pondicherry, India [35].
Saxena et al [36]	Saxena et al reported on entomological investigations of Japanese encephalitis outbreak in Gorakhpur and Deoria districts of Uttar Pradesh, India [36].
Sharma et al [37]	Sharma et al reported on clinical profile of the Japanese encephalitis epidemics in Goa in 1982-1983 [37].
Chakrabarty et al [38]	Chakrabarty et al reported on epidemiological investigations of Japanese encephalitis outbreak in Gorakhpur and Deoria districts of Uttar Pradesh 1985 [38] .
Chakrabarty et al [39]	Chakraborty et al reported on an outbreak of Japanese encephalitis in Manipur during 1982 focusing on some epidemiological features [39].
Mohan Rao et al [40]	Mohan Rao et al descried for the first laboratory proven outbreak of Japanese encephalitis in Goa [40].
Shankar et al [41]	Shankar et al described for autopsy study of brains during an epidemic of Japanese encephalitis in Karnataka, India [41].
Biswas et al [42]	Biswas et al reported on epidemic of Japanese encephalitis in Bankura in 1973 focusing on clinico-pathological findings [42].
Rodrigues et al [43]	Rodrigues et al reported on the 1973 epidemic of Japanese encephalitis in West Bengal by a serological survey of domestic animals [43].
Mukherji and Biswas [44]	Mukherji and Biswas reported on Histopathological studies of brains and other viscera from cases of Japanese encephalitis during 1973 epidemic at Bankura, India [44].
Sen Gupta et al [45]	Sen Gupta et al reported on clinical profile of the epidemic of Japanese encephalitis at Bankura, India [45].
Rajagopalan and Panicker [46]	Rajagopalan and Panicker decribed a note on the 1976 epidemic of Japanese encephalitis in Burdwan district, West Bengal, India [46].
Rao et al [47]	Rao et al reported on investigations of the 1978 epidemic of encephalitis in Asansol, West Bengal and Dhanbad, Bihar, India [47].

1. Japanese Encephalitis in India

India is a big country. There are also some areas that lie in the tropical region. Therefore, the problem of Japanese encephalitis can be seen. Japanese encephalitis can be classified as an important emerging infection in India. There are many reports on the emergence of Japanese encephalitis in India as shown in Table 1.

2. Japanese Encephalitis in Nepal

Nepal is another country in South Asia. There are no reports on the emergence of Japanese encephalitis in Nepal. This might be due to the fact that Nepal is not in the tropical area of Asia.

3. Japanese Encephalitis in Bhutan

Bhutan is another country in South Asia. There are no reports on the emergence of Japanese encephalitis in Bhutan. This might be due to the fact that Bhutan is not in the tropical area of Asia.

4. Japanese Encephalitis in Maldives

Maldives is another country in South Asia. Of interest, there are no reports on the emergence of Japanese encephalitis in Maldives although this country lies in tropical zone. This may be due to the fact that this country is a combination of several islands in the Indian ocean.

5. Japanese Encephalitis in Sri Lanka

Sri Lanka is another country in South Asia. There are some interesting reports on the outbreaks or epidemics of Japanese encephalitis in Sri Lanka. Peiris et al reported on an outbreak of Japanese encephalitis in Sri Lanka [48]. Peiris et al performed a prospective study of mosquito vectors, porcine infection and human disease during a Japanese encephalitis (JE) epidemic in the North Central province of Sri Lanka (November-December 1987) and a subsequent non-epidemic year (1988) and reported that the main difference between the epidemic (1987) and non-epidemic (1988) years was a lower vector biomass and lower rates of virus carriage in the mosquito population [48].

6. Japanese Encephalitis in Bangladesh

Bangladesh is another country in South Asia. There are some interesting reports on the outbreaks or epidemics of Japanese encephalitis in Bangladesh. Khan et al described a focus of Japanese encephalitis in the Modhupur Forest area; Bangladesh and mentioned that this disease was diagnosed for the first time in Bangladesh [49]. In this work [49], the diagnosis was based on the clinical appearance of the disease and the results of serological investigations [49].

7. Japanese encephalitis in Pakistan

Pakistan is another country in South Asia. However, there is no report on the emergence of Japanese encephalitis in Pakistan.

The Emergence of other Arboviruses in South Asia

1. West Nile Virus Infection

The West Nile virus infection is a new emerging infectious disease in many areas of the world. The clinical presentation is high fever and ends with deadly encephalitis. Morbidity and mortality due to this infection is very high. West Nile virus infection is not common in South Asia although it is a problematic emerging infection in other areas of the world. There is no outbreak of this disease. However, there is an interesting report. Sugamata reported on dependence on the birth season of the antibody level against West Nile virus in the Pakistani population [50]. Sugamata noted that the ability to produce antibodies against WN virus among Pakistani persons might depend on their birth season [50].

2. Chandipura Virus Encephalitis

Chandipura virus encephalitis is an important emerging infectious disease first reported in India (Table 2).

This virus infection is mentioned as a new emerging infection in India [53]. Andhra Pradesh was the first identified setting. Tandale et al said that this viral infection was the major cause of acute viral encephalitis in children in endemic areas during early monsoon months [54]. Acute encephalitis is the main presentation and serological diagnosis is useful.

Table 2. Reports on the emergence of Chandipura virus encephalitis in India.

Author	Details
Chadha et al [51]	Chadha et al reported on an outbreak of Chandipura virus encephalitis in the eastern districts of Gujarat state, India [51].
Rao et al [52]	Rao et al reported on a large outbreak of acute encephalitis with high fatality rate in children in Andhra Pradesh, India, in 2003, associated with Chandipura virus [52].

References

[1] Halstead SB, Jacobson J. Japanese encephalitis. *Adv Virus Res*. 2003; 61: 103-38

[2] Solomon T. Exotic and emerging viral encephalitides. *Curr Opin Neurol.* 2003; 16: 411-8.

[3] Whitley RJ, Gnann JW. Viral encephalitis: familiar infections and emerging pathogens. *Lancet.* 2002; 359: 507-13.

[4] Mackenzie JS, Gubler DJ, Petersen LR. Emerging flaviviruses: the spread and resurgence of Japanese encephalitis, West Nile and dengue viruses. *Nat Med* 2004; 10(12 Suppl): S98-S109.

[5] Gubler DJ. The global emergence/resurgence of arboviral diseases as public health problems. *Arch Med Res*. 2002; 33: 330-42.

[6] Zeller HG. Dengue, arbovirus and migrations in the Indian Ocean. *Bull Soc Pathol Exot.* 1998; 91: 56-60.

[7] Wiwanitkit V. Amazing Thailand Year 1998-1999 Tourist's health concepts. *Chula Med J.* 1998; 42: 975-984.

[8] Bucens M, O'Connor L. Japanese encephalitis and the traveller. *Aust Fam Physician*. 1990; 19: 163-5.

[9] King NJ, Shrestha B, Kesson AM. Immune modulation by flaviviruses. *Adv Virus Res*. 2003; 60: 121-55.

[10] Kanojia PC, Jamgaonkar AV. Mosquito records from a hot and dry climatic area experiencing frequent outbreaks of Japanese encephalitis, Bellary district, Karnataka, India. *J Am Mosq Control Assoc*. 2008 Mar;24(1):6-10.

[11] Gupta N, Chatterjee K, Karmakar S, Jain SK, Venkatesh S, Lal S. Bellary, India achieves negligible case fatality due to Japanese encephalitis despite no vaccination: an outbreak investigation in 2004. *Indian J Pediatr*. 2008 Jan;75(1):31-7.

[12] Parida M, Dash PK, Tripathi NK, Ambuj, Sannarangaiah S, Saxena P, Agarwal S, Sahni AK, Singh SP, Rathi AK, Bhargava R, Abhyankar A, Verma SK, Rao PV, Sekhar K. Japanese Encephalitis Outbreak, India, 2005. *Emerg Infect Dis*. 2006 Sep;12(9):1427-30.

[13] Lawrence J. Japanese encephalitis outbreak in India and Nepal. *Euro Surveill*. 2005 Sep 22;10(9):E050922.4.

[14] Kumar R, Tripathi P, Singh S, Bannerji G. Clinical features in children hospitalized during the 2005 epidemic of Japanese encephalitis in Uttar Pradesh, *India. Clin Infect Dis*. 2006 Jul 15;43(2):123-31.

[15] Gupta N, Hossain S, Lal R, Das BP, Venkatesh S, Chatterjee K. Epidemiological profile of Japanese encephalitis outbreak in Gorakhpur, UP in 2004. *J Commun Dis*. 2005 Jun;37(2):145

[16] Rao P, Joshi K, Mishra B, Ratho RK, Kumar R. An outbreak of Japanese encephalitis in Haryana. *J Commun Dis*. 2005 Mar;37(1):78-81.

[17] Mudur G. Japanese encephalitis outbreak kills 1300 children in India. *BMJ*. 2005 Dec 3;331(7528):1288

[18] Chatterjee P. Japanese encephalitis outbreak in India. *Lancet Neurol*. 2005 Nov;4(11):700.

[19] Raut CG, Thakare JP, Padbidri VS, Sapkal GN, Mishra AC, Paramasivan R, Gokhale MD, Mourya DT, Shouche YS, Jayakumar PC. A focal outbreak of Japanese Encephalitis among horses in Pune district, India. *J Commun Dis*. 2003 Mar;35(1):40-2.

[20] Kaur R, Agarwal CS, Das D. An investigation into the JE epidemic of 2000 in Upper Assam--a perspective study. *J Commun Dis*. 2002 Jun;34(2):135-45.

[21] Arunachalam N, Philip Samuel P, Hiriyan J, Thenmozhi V, Balasubramanian A, Gajanana A, Satyanarayana K. Vertical transmission of Japanese encephalitis virus in Mansonia species, in an epidemic-prone area of southern India. *Ann Trop Med Parasitol*. 2002 Jun;96(4):419-20.

[22] Rao JS, Misra SP, Patanayak SK, Rao TV, Das Gupta RK, Thapar BR. Japanese Encephalitis epidemic in Anantapur district, Andhra Pradesh (October-November, 1999). *J Commun Dis*. 2000 Dec;32(4):306-12.

[23] Dash AP, Chhotray GP, Mahapatra N, Hazra RK. Retrospective analysis of epidemiological investigation of Japanese encephalitis outbreak occurred in Rourkela, Orissa, India. *Southeast Asian J Trop Med Public Health*. 2001 Mar;32(1):137-9.

[24] Outbreak news. Japanese encephalitis, India. *Wkly Epidemiol Rec*. 1999 Dec 17;74(50):440.

[25] Neogi DK, Bhattacharya N, Chakrabarti T, Mukherjee KK. Detection of HIV seropositivity during an outbreak of Japanese encephalitis in Manipur. *J Commun Dis*. 1998 Jun;30(2):113-6.

[26] Dhanda V, Thenmozhi V, Kumar NP, Hiriyan J, Arunachalam N, Balasubramanian A, Ilango A, Gajanana A. Virus isolation from wild-caught mosquitoes during a Japanese encephalitis outbreak in Kerala in 1996. *Indian J Med Res*. 1997 Jul;106:4-6.

[27] Rathi AK, Kushwaha KP, Singh YD, Singh J, Sirohi R, Singh RK, Singh UK. JE virus encephalitis: 1988 epidemic at Gorakhpur. *Indian Pediatr*. 1993 Mar;30(3):325-33.

[28] Vajpayee A, Dey PN, Chakraborty AK, Chakraborty MS. Study of the outbreak of Japanese encephalitis in Lakhimpur district of Assam in 1989. *J Indian Med Assoc*. 1992 May;90(5):114-5.

[29] Sharma SN, Panwar BS. An epidemic of Japanese encephalitis in Haryana in the year 1990. *J Commun Dis*. 1991 Sep;23(3):204-5.

[30] Sharma RC, Saxena VK, Bharadwaj M, Sharma RS, Verghese T, Datta KK. An outbreak of Japanese encephalitis in Haryana--1990. *J Commun Dis.* 1991 Jun;23(2):168-9.

[31] Vajpayee A, Mukherjee MK, Chakraborty AK, Chakraborty MS. Investigation of an outbreak of Japanese encephalitis in Rourkela City (Orissa) during 1989. *J Commun Dis.* 1991 Mar;23(1):18-21.

[32] Mukherjee KK, Chakravarti SK, Mukherjee MK, De PN, Chatterjee S, Chatterjee P, Chakraborty MS. Recurrent outbreaks of Japanese encephalitis in Nagaland (1985-1989)--a seroepidemiological study. *J Commun Dis.* 1991 Mar;23(1):11-7.

[33] Narasimham MV, Rao CK, Bendle MS, Yadava RL, Johri YC, Pandey RS. Epidemiological investigation on Japanese encephalitis outbreak in Uttar Pradesh during 1988. *J Commun Dis.* 1988 Dec;20(4):263-75.

[34] Chakraborty AK, Chakravarti SK, Chakravarty MS. Outbreak of Japanese encephalitis in two districts of Assam during 1980: some epidemiological features. *Indian J Public Health.* 1987 Jan-Mar;31(1):5-11

[35] Rao CV, Risbud AR, Rodrigues FM, Pinto BD, Joshi GD. The 1981 epidemic of Japanese encephalitis in Tamil Nadu & Pondicherry. *Indian J Med Res.* 1988 May;87:417-21.

[36] Saxena VK, Baig MH, Bhardwaj M, Rajagopal R. Entomological investigations of Japanese encephalitis outbreak in Gorakhpur and Deoria districts of Uttar Pradesh. *J Commun Dis.* 1986 Sep;18(3):219-21

[37] Sharma NG, Dubhashi NG, Mohandas KM, Pereira P. Clinical profile of the Japanese encephalitis epidemics in Goa in 1982-83. J Assoc Physicians India. 1985 Dec;33(12):767-9, 771.

[38] Chakrabarty S, Saxena VK, Bhardwaj M. Epidemiological investigations of Japanese encephalitis outbreak in Gorakhpur and Deoria districts of Uttar Pradesh 1985. *J Commun Dis.* 1986 Jun;18(2):103-8.

[39] Chakraborty AK, Chakraborty SK, Chakraborty MS, Singh NC. Outbreak of Japanese encephalitis in Manipur during 1982--some epidemiological features. *J Commun Dis.* 1984 Sep;16(3):227-33.

[40] Mohan Rao CV, Prasad SR, Rodrigues JJ, Sharma NG, Shaikh BH, Pavri KM. The first laboratory proven outbreak of Japanese encephalitis in Goa. *Indian J Med Res.* 1983 Dec;78:745-50.

[41] Shankar SK, Rao TV, Mruthyunjayanna BP, Gourie Devi M, Deshpande DH. Autopsy study of brains during an epidemic of Japanese encephalitis in Karnataka. *Indian J Med Res.* 1983 Sep;78:431-40

[42] Biswas SK, Bose SN, Bose M, Roychoudhury D, Nundy NK, Mukherji S, Saha SC, Sarkar R, Banerji N, Chatterji R. Epidemic of Japanese encephalitis in Bankura (1973): clinico-pathological findings. *Indian J Med Res.* 1976 Jun;64(6):801-7

[43] Rodrigues FM, Vidyasagar J, Singh PB, Ghosh SN, Guttikar SN, Joshi MV, Gupta NP. The 1973 epidemic of Japanese encephalitis in West Bengal: a serological survey of domestic animals. *Indian J Med Res.* 1976 Jul;64(7):973-80

[44] Mukherji AK, Biswas SK. Histopathological studies of brains (and other viscera) from cases of JE virus encephalitis during 1973 epidemic at Bankura. *Indian J Med Res.* 1976 Aug;64(8):1143-9.

[45] Sen Gupta SN, Sen MK, Das PK, Bhattacharya DP, Rath BB. Clinical profile of the epidemic of Japanese encephalitis at Bankura. *Indian J Med Res.* 1976 Oct;64(10):1393-402.

[46] Rajagopalan PK, Panicker KN. A note on the 1976 epidemic of Japanese encephalitis in Burdwan district, West Bengal. *Indian J Med Res.* 1978 Sep;68:3938.

[47] Rao CV, Banerjee K, Mandke VB, Dandawate CN, Ilkal MA, Anand BR, Biswas PN, Ray M. Investigations of the 1978 epidemic of encephalitis in Asansol, West Bengal and Dhanbad, Bihar. *J Assoc Physicians India.* 1980 Nov;28(11):441-9.

[48] Peiris JS, Amerasinghe FP, Amerasinghe PH, Ratnayake CB, Karunaratne SH, Tsai TF. Japanese encephalitis in Sri Lanka--the study of an epidemic: vector incrimination, porcine infection and human disease. *Trans R Soc Trop Med Hyg.* 1992 May-Jun;86(3):307-13.

[49] Khan AM, Khan AQ, Dobrzynski L, Joshi GP, Myat A. A Japanese encephalitis focus in Bangladesh. *J Trop Med Hyg.* 1981 Feb;84(1):41-4.

[50] Sugamata M. Dependence on the birth season of the antibody level against West Nile virus in the Pakistani population. *Acta Virol.* 1988 Mar;32(2):138-47.

[51] Chadha MS, Arankalle VA, Jadi RS, Joshi MV, Thakare JP, Mahadev PV, Mishra AC. An outbreak of Chandipura virus encephalitis in the eastern districts of Gujarat state, India. *Am J Trop Med Hyg.* 2005 Sep;73(3):566-70.

[52] Rao BL, Basu A, Wairagkar NS, Gore MM, Arankalle VA, Thakare JP, Jadi RS, Rao KA, Mishra AC. A large outbreak of acute encephalitis with high fatality rate in children in Andhra Pradesh, India, in 2003, associated with Chandipura virus. *Lancet.* 2004 Sep 4-10;364(9437):869-74.

[53] Van Ranst M. Chandipura virus: an emerging human pathogen? *Lancet.* 2004 Sep 4-10;364(9437):821-2.

[54] Tandale BV, Tikute SS, Arankalle VA, Sathe PS, Joshi MV, Ranadive SN, Kanojia PC, Eshwarachary D, Kumarswamy M, Mishra AC. Chandipura virus: a major cause of acute encephalitis in children in North Telangana, Andhra Pradesh, *India. J Med Virol.* 2008 Jan;80(1):118-24.

Chapter VIII

Gastrointestinal Infectious Disease in India

Gastrointestinal Infection in India: An Existing Problem

India is a developing country in Asia with high prevalence of gastrointestinal infection. As already mentioned in the first chapter, India can also be expressed as a subcontinent of Asia covering many countries that combine to form South Asia. Many specific cultures of India, which are presently well known, exist. This is considered to be the world's oldest rooted culture which affects the lifestyle of the Indian and has several effects on health. Due to the highly populated characteristics, India has many public health problems. This is the common cause of communicable disease in India. For sure, these gastrointestinal infectious diseases can cause very high mortality and morbidity. Also, there are many emerging and reemerging gastrointestinal infectious diseases in India. The specific aim of this chapter is to focus on those emerging and reemerging gastrointestinal infectious diseases in India.

Outbreak and Transmission of Gastrointestinal Infection

By easy definition, gastrointestinal infection can mean infection that occurs within gastrointestinal tract, especially the stomach, small intestine and large intestine. There are several kinds of gastrointestinal infections. It should be noted that gastrointestinal infection is common because of the fact that everybody has to eat food and so everyone enters a foreign body into the gastrointestinal tract via mouth everyday and these foreign bodies can be contaminated by pathogenic organisms. Talking about pathogenic organisms, the bacteria pathogens seems to be the most important group. There are several problematic gastrointestinal bacteria that cause gastrointestinal infections. In addition to bacteria, the parasite is another common group of pathogens that can cause gastrointestinal infection. This infection is specifically called a gastrointestinal parasitic infestation.

"You are what you eat" can be the best description for the scenario of gastrointestinal infection. Because the main route of transmission of gastrointestinal infection is oral ingestion, the sanitation of food is the most concerning topic in the management of gastrointestinal infection. The so called feco-oral route makes it seem that the ones who get gastrointestinal infections have to eat contaminated food that carried another's feces. This is a very big problem of many developing countries especially for India and nearby countries in South Asia. Considering the pathway, the infected person passes the contaminated feces into the environment by poor toilet habit. This is the main focus for toilet sanitation. Others can make contact with the contaminated feces via several means. This can be due to dirty hand grasping food, contamination in vegetables, etc. In many developing countries, feces are used as fertilizer for growing vegetables. Some may also get infection by the ingestion of rare or poorly cooked food that is already contaminated by an infected person. Mostly, contaminated food is eaten and causes the gastrointestinal infection. This seems simple but really occurs. Focusing on the pathway, there are many steps to be mentioned. Poor toilet habits are the first step to be mentioned. Toileting must be performed with a well-designed place to control the spreading of contaminated feces. The problem in any rural ares of developing countries is the fact that the local people usually do not use the toilet. They pass their excreta in the field directly and can be the source for spreading of the pathogenic organism. The second thing to be mentioned are the eating habits. Eating is the basic human activity. However, sanitation for eating is needed yet is usually problematic. Everybody has to eat with proper sanitation in mind. Hand washing before eating and cooking food well are the two basic principles. In addition, the utensil used for cooking and eating has to be clean. Local people should be taught not to eat poorly cooked food because it can cause infection. Contamination within the food can be effectively managed by heat. This is the basic concept. The ones who eat well cooked food have more safety than the ones who do not. This can confirm the fact that "you are what you eat."

Contamination by germs during cooking is the biggest problem and can bring the outbreak of gastrointestinal infection. The cause of many outbreaks is due to the common source of contamination by a cook. The cook is the one who prepares the food for large groups of people therefore he/she has to have the good sanitation in cooking food and has to be screened for infection. Water is another point to be concerned. Water can be contaminated. Everyone has to drink water to maintain their physiological process. Contaminated water is the root cause of many outbreaks. In India, there are many reported gastrointestinal infection outbreaks due to contaminated water. Similar to food, ones who prepare drinks for a large group of people has to be controlled for health status and sanitation. Outbreak due to contamination of food and water should be managed and can be managed by basic sanitation promotion. In the scenario of India, the food and water borne disease is still an important public health problem to be managed. Some details on important diseases will be further shown in this chapter.

Malarial Diarrhea

Introduction

Diarrhea is a common gastrointestinal disorder. Several causes of diarrhea can be seen. However, there can be some rare causes of diarrhea including malaria. Malarial infection is an important tropical infectious disease that is caused by a mosquito bite. Many rural populations in the tropical zone are at risk for this infection. The infection usually has classical symptoms such as fever and chill [1]. However, there are also other unusual manifestations of this tropical infection [1]. An important unusual manifestation of malaria is diarrhea. In this brief review, the author will briefly review on diarrhea in malarial infection.

Magnitude of the Problem

There are several documented rare manifestations of malaria. This includes the case of diarrhea. According to a previous publication by Suyaphan et al [1], the incidence of diarrhea in the cases with malaria was equal to 3.3 %. A similar high prevalence (5 %) was also reported by Zaher et al [3]. The reported rates are considerably high and require an interest in gastroenterology. Concerning the pattern of diarrhea, watery diarrhea was common [1].

Pathogenesis and Pathology

The root cause of diarrhea in malaria is not well known. Some mentioned that this might be only a co-presentation. The poor sanitation in the endemic area of malaria can bring the vulnerability to diarrhea [4 - 5]. However, there is some evidence indicating that malaria can directly cause diarrhea [6]. Reisinger et al said that intestinal villi disturbance due to the malarial parasite induced ischemia and is the main pathogenesis of malarial diarrhea [7]. Molyneux et al noted that malabsorption of sugars, amino acids and fats could be seen due to this pathology [8]. Wilairatana et al noted that the described increased gastrointestinal permeability were significant in patients with Plasmodium falciparum malaria [9]. Prasad and Virk mentioned that these processes contributed to the pathogenesis of watery diarrhea in malaria [10]. Reisinger et al also noted that malara with such severe diarrhea met the WHO criteria for complicated malaria and had an increased mortality rate [7]. However, there were no associations between diarrhea and parasite rate, parasite density, or clinical malaria [11].

Diarrhea Due to Antimalarial Drug

In addition to the malaria parasite, diarrhea can be the result of the antimalarial drug. There are some reports on this topic for mefloquine, a classical antimalarial drug.

Luxembergur et al reported that the significant side effect of mefloquine is gastrointestinal disturbance [12]. Diarrhea can be seen [12]. However, ter Kuile et al said that this side effect of mefloquine was not serious [13]. Concerning the new antimalarial drug artesunate, Luxembergur et al found that there was no gastrointestinal side effect [12]. Many other reports also confirm this finding [14 – 17]. Concerning the combination, artesunate and mefloquine, the rate of diarrhea can be seen in 0 – 16 % [17].

Therapeutic Concern

As previously mentioned, malarial diarrhea can be severe. The treatment of diarrhea in malaria is usually symptomatic. In severe cases presenting with severe dehydration, intravenous fluid administration can be selected. However, the important point is that it is necessary to make early diagnosis and give prompt treatment for the baseline etiology, the malarial infection. Exclusion for the other possible treatable causes of diarrhea is needed.

Typhoid Fever

Introduction to Typhoid Fever

Typhoid is another important bacterial gastrointestinal infection. This basterail infection is noted as an important food borne disease and *Salmonella* spp is the main pathogen. Considering the pathophysiology, a strong host innate immune/inflammatory response induction plays important pathophysiological roles. It is not well explained if this ultimately shows an adaptive advantage to the host or pathogenic organism [18]. Typhoid fever hits averagely 20 million human beings annually and causes at least 700,000 mortalities [19]. The main burden of the disease is in several developing tropical countries including India [19]. Concerning the presentation of typhoid fever in clinics, high fever with diarrhea is usually detected. Considering the pathology, the ileum is the main affected organ. A case series from Taiwan showed the most common complaints of the patients with typhoid fever were fever, diarrhea, abdominal pain, and cough [20]. Relative bradycardia and leucopenia were also commonly described laboratory results [20]. For diagnosis of typhoid fever, the Widal test is a very classical and well-known serological laboratory test [21]. Although this serological test was approved for a century as a serologic means of determining the existence of typhoid fever the Widal test continues to be controversial owing to the limited quality of the antigens used and the interpretation of the laboratory results [22].

Typhoid Fever in India

Typhoid fever is still endemic in India. There are some reports on the prevalence of typhoid fever in India. John said that typhoid fever was one of the focused emerging infectious diseases in India [23]. Jog et al studied on typhoid fever in Mumbai, India [24]. They found that high culture positivity despite prior or ongoing antibiotic treatment was seen and an absolute eosinophil count of 0% could be an important marker of typhoid [24]. A high prevalence of nalidixic acid resistance was also reported in this paper [24]. Patil et al studied baseline Widal titres in healthy Indian children and reported that the baseline titres for either *S. enterica* subsp. enterica ser. Typhi antigen in 6 month-2 year was equal to 1:40 and older children was equal to 1:80 whereas the baseline titres for H antigen of *S. enterica* subsp. enterica ser. Paratyphi A in 0.5-2 year was less than 1:20 and for older children was equal to 1:40 dilution [25]. Of interest, Dutta et al noted an emergence of highly fluoroquinolone-resistant *S. enterica* serovar Typhi in community-based fever surveillance from Kolkata, India [26].

Table 1. Reports on the emergenceof typhoid fever in India.

Author	Details
Palit et al [27]	Palit et al reported on increasing prevalence of *S. enterica* serotype Paratyphi-A in patients with enteric fever in a periurban slum setting of Kolkata, India [27].
Woods et al [28]	Woods et al reported on emergence of *S. enterica* serotype Paratyphi A as a major cause of enteric fever in Kathmandu, Nepal [28].
Lakshmi et al [29]	Lakshmi et al reported on increasing prevalence of resistant Salmonella isolates at a tertiary care hospital in Hyderabad , India [29].
Mandal et al [30]	Mandal et al reported on increased prevalence of antibiotic resistance of *S. enterica* serovar Paratyphi A in India [30].

For treatment of typhoid fever in India, the therapeutic protocol must be adapted responding to the increasing drug resistance problem. As a recommendation, Manchanda et al said that "there is an urgent need for further clinical studies to evaluate response to chloramphenicol in such cases. Antimicrobial susceptibility data and MIC distribution favour use of ampicillin as a drug of choice for the treatment of enteric fever.[31]" Manchanda et al noted that third generation cephalosporins were another useful alternative but the usage of third generation cephalosporins should be restricted for complicated cases [31].

For prevention of typhoid fever, water sanitation and immunization in the existence of gross generalized antibiotic resistance in India is the focused activity [32 - 33]. However, vaccination against typhoid fever is still another important tool for the key point of management of this disease. In the present day, there are at least two commercial vaccines for typhoid fever in clinical practice. One is based on defined subunit virulence polysaccharide antigen and can be injected either intramuscularly or subcutaneously, the other is live attenuated vaccine that can be orally administrated. At present, typhoid vaccination is recommended for any travelers planning a visit to moderate- to high-risk tropical countries including India [32 - 33]. However, an important contraindication for typhoid vaccination is for human immunodeficiency virus (HIV) infected vaccinees [34]. Levine mentioned that partnerships of public and private agencies in the developing and the industrialized countries helped create a reliable demand for reliable typhoid vaccines in order to confirm adequate, sustained supplies of affordably produced vaccines [35]. Concerning the side effect of the typhoid vaccine, it is considered not dangerous [32 – 33]. However, there are some considerable rare adverse effects such as encephalitis [36]. As far as minor tolerable adverse effects go, metabolic and febrile adverse effects to the typhoid vaccine, owing to the effect of beta-adrenergic blockade, are documented in the literature [37].

Cholera

Introduction to Cholera

Cholera is an important bacterial diarrhea with long history. There have been many outbreaks in world history causing millions of death. It is classified as a severe watery diarrhea transmitted by the feco-oral route bacterial infection and is strongly related to poverty and poor sanitation [38]. Every year, more than 100,000 cholera cases are reported and 2,000-3,000 mortalities are noted [39]. The real figures for cholera are thought to be much higher due to underreporting and lack of good surveillance systems [39]. Cholera is generated by a gram-negative bacterium, *Vibrio cholera* pathogen [39]. The diagnosis of cholera can be made by the clinical appearance and confirmed by the microbiological examination. The routine bacterial culture can be helpful. A simple basic investigation tool is the fresh smear to detect the shooting star appearance of the pathogenic organism. Presently, many tropical countries, especially India and Bangladesh, are considered endemic areas for cholera [40].

Cholera in India

There are many reports on cholera from India. As already said India is a well known endemic area of cholera. There are many root behaviors preventing the promotion of good sanitation in India. One of the important root beliefs to be mentioned is the delivery of the dead bodies into the river hoping that this will bring the dead to the heaven. This can bring the infectious disease to the ones who use water from that river. There are many reports on outbreaks and emergences of cholera from India as shown in Table 1. For cholera, many putative virulence genes of *Vibrio cholerae* from seafood and the coastal environment of India were reported [41]. Das et al noted that there was a new trend of antibiotic resistance of *Vibrio cholerae* strains from East Delhi, India [42]. This can be a big problem. Reports on the emergence of cholera in India are shown in Table 2.

For treatment of cholera, the basic fluid management is needed. However, antibiotics should be administered in the cases with invasive characteristics. The important problem to be concerned with is the antibiotic resistance cholera. For prevention, similar to typhoid fever, water sanitation is the main means for cholera control because almost all past outbreaks of cholera in India were owing to the water contamination. Griffith et al reported that the most significant risk factors were water contamination by the pathogen, heavy rainfall and flooding, and population dislocation [51]. However, owing to the good running tap water at present, the outbreak of cholera can be successfully reduced in many developing countries but not India. For prevention, a cholera vaccine is available. Large-scale field trials have readily confirmed the efficacy and safety of the oral cholera vaccine in various forms [52]. For travelers, certain higher risk groups who wanted to visit India might benefit from prevention against cholera by vaccination [52 - 55]. Basically, cholera-killing whole cell vaccines are effective and safe and recommended. Its protection appears to persist up to 24 months following a single dose of the vaccine, and for three to four years with an annual booster [56]. However, Lopez et al pointed out that although internationally available, oral cholera vaccines were not widely used in public health settings in developing countries where the vaccines were highly required for medical usage [54]. A successful subunit cholera vaccine that can provide protective immunity with one parenteral immunization is the new aim for replacing the classical oral vaccines that have two doses for optimal prevention [52 - 55]. However, owing to decision analysis, routine vaccination of travelers to endemic areas, especially for India, is still recommended [57].

Table 2. Reports on the emergence of cholera in India.

Author	Details
Shukla and Alam [43]	Shukla and Alam reported on emergence of *Vibrio cholerae* OI biotype EIT or serotype Inaba in Aligarh [43].
Rajeshwari et al [44]	Rajeshwari et al reported on diarrheal outbreak of *Vibrio cholerae* 01 Inaba in Delhi [44].
Khuntia et al [45]	Khuntia et al reported that environmental *Vibrio cholerae* O139 might be the progenitor of outbreak of cholera in coastal area of Orissa, eastern India, 2000: molecular evidence [45].
Pal et al [46]	Pal et al reported on emergence of Vibrio cholerae O1 biotype El Tor serotype Inaba causing outbreaks of cholera in Orissa, India [46].
Roychowdhury et al [47]	Roychowdhury et al reported on emergence of tetracycline-resistant Vibrio cholerae O1 serotype Inaba, in Kolkata, India [47].
Gupta et al [48]	Gupta et al reported on an el tor cholera outbreak amongst tribal population in Tripura, India [48].
Taneja et al [49]	Taneja et al reported on emergence of *Vibrio cholerae* O1 Biotype El Tor serotype Inaba in north India [49].
Gomber et al [50]	Gomber et al reported on diarrheal outbreak of Vibrio cholerae 0139 from north India [50].

Shigellosis

Shigellosis is another important bacterial infection. This is classified as an invasive bacterial diarrhea. Affected cases will pass bloody stool [58]. Bloody diarrhea makes this infection different from watery diarrhea in cholera. Four species of Shigella including *S. dysenteriae*, *S. flexneri*, *S. boydii* and *S. sonnei* have the ability to cause the disease [58]. These problematic species can be subdivided into serotypes on the basis of O-specific polysaccharide of the LPS [58]. *S. dysenteriae* type 1 produces severe disease and may bring life-threatening complications [58].

For diagnosis, culturing the stool samples using selective/differential agar media is the recommendation [58]. The diagnosis of shigellosis can be made by the clinical appearance and confirmed by the microbiological test. The routine bacterial culture can be useful. Shigella spp. are highly fragile organisms and considerable care must be used in collecting fecal specimens, transporting them to the laboratories and in using appropriate media for isolation. Similar to other gastrointestinal diseases, shigellosis is still problematic in India. This is a concern for public health in India [59 – 60]. There are many reports on the emergence of shigellosis in India as briefly summarized in Table 3.

Table 3. Reports on the emergence of shigellosis in India.

Author	Details
Niyogi et al [61]	Niyogi et al reported on an outbreak of bacillary dysentery caused by quinolone-resistant Shigella dysenteriae type 1 in a northeastern state of India [61].
Singh et al [62]	Singh et al reported on an outbreak of shigellosis in a slum colony of Delhi-1990 [62].
Sengupta et al [63]	Sengupta et al reported on a multidrug resistant epidemic shigellosis in a village in west Bengal, 1984 [63].
Datta and Sen [64]	Datta and Sen reported on an outbreak of dysentery due to nalidixic acid resistant *S. dysenteriae* 1 at Agartala, Tripura, India [64].

For treatment of shigellosis, similar to other gastrointestinal infectious disease, basic fluid management is needed. In addition, antibiotics should be administered in the cases with invasive characteristics. The important problem to be concerned with is the antibiotic resistant shigellosis. For prevention, similar to other gastrointestinal infectious diseases, water sanitation is the main means for shigellosis control because almost all past outbreaks of shigellosis in India were due to the water contamination.

Poliomyelitis

Poliomyelitis is a viral infectious disease that causes high rates of disability. Motor paralysis is the important complication of this infection. The transmission of poliomylelitis is due to the oro-fecal route [65 – 66]. Poor sanitation is believed to be the main factor contributing to this serious viral infection. There are some interesting reports on the emergence of shigellosis in India as briefly summarized in Table 4.

Table 4. Reports on the emergence of poliomyelitis in India.

Author	Details
Mandke et al [67]	Mandke et al reported on an outbreak of poliomyelitis in the Marathwada region of Maharashtra State, India [67].
Murthy et al [68]	Murthy et al reported on outbreak of poliomyelitis in Andhra Pradesh, South India [68].
Wadia et al [69]	Wadia et al reported on polio-like motor paralysis associated with acute hemorrhagic conjunctivitis in an outbreak in 1981 in Bombay, India [69].
Lowalekar et al [70]	Lowalekar et al reported on an epidemic of polio-like neuroparalytic disease associated with acute haemorrhagic conjunctivitis in India [70].
Chakraborty et al [71]	Chakraborty et al reported on an outbreak of poliomyelitis in Alleppey town, Kerala, India [71].
Sundaravalli [72]	Sundaravalli reported on spurts of poliomyelitis in Madras, India [72].
Saeed et al [73]	Saeed et al reported on an outbreak of poliomyelitis in Allahabad, India [73].
Agarwal and Agarwal [74]	Agarwal and Agarwal reported on their observations on a recent outbreak of poliomyelitis in Allahabad, India [74].

Poliomyelitis is a disease of present focus. The attempt to increase the coverage of the polio vaccine seems to be the tool to reach the aim of eradication of this disease from India [75 – 77].

References

[1] Suyaphun A, Wiwanitkit V, Suwansaksri J, Nithiuthai S, Sritar S, Suksirisampant W, Fongsungnern A. Malaria among hilltribe communities in northern Thailand: a review of clinical manifestations. *Southeast Asian J Trop Med Public Health.* 2002;33 Suppl 3:14-5.

[2] Wiwanitkit V. Overt bleeding in malarial patients: experience and review. *Blood Coagul Fibrinolysis.* 2008 Jan;19(1):1-4.

[3] Zaher T, Ahmadi M, Ibrahim A, El-Bahnasawy M, Gouda H, Shahat SA. Malaria in Egypt, Saudi Arabia and Yemen: a clinical pilot study. *J Egypt Soc Parasitol.* 2007 Dec;37(3):969-76.

[4] House HR, Ehlers JP. Travel-related infections. *Emerg Med Clin North Am.* 2008 May;26(2):499-516, x.

[5] Kaler SG. Diseases of poverty with high mortality in infants and children: malaria, measles, lower respiratory infections, and diarrheal illnesses. *Ann N Y Acad Sci.* 2008;1136:28-31.

[6] Schulthess G, Kolyvanos Naumann U, Käser L, Vetter W. Malaria. Primary symptoms: fever, headache, nausea, vomiting, diarrhea. *Praxis* (Bern 1994). 2006 Feb 22;95(8):255-60.

[7] Reisinger EC, Fritzsche C, Krause R, Krejs GJ. Diarrhea caused by primarily non-gastrointestinal infections. *Nat Clin Pract Gastroenterol Hepatol.* 2005 May;2(5):216-22.

[8] Molyneux ME, Looareesuwan S, Menzies IS, Grainger SL, Phillips RE, Wattanagoon Y, Thompson RP, Warrell DA. Reduced hepatic flow and intestinal malabsorption in severe falciparum malaria. *Am J Trop Med Hyg* 1989 May;40(5):470-6.

[9] Wilairatana P, Meddings JB, Ho M, Vannaphan S, Looareesuwan S. Increased gastrointestinal permeability in patients with Plasmodium falciparum malaria. *Clin Infect Dis.* 1997 Mar; 24(3): 430–435.

[10] Prasad NR, Virk KJ. Malaria as a cause of diarrhoea - a review. *N G Med J.* 1993 Dec;36(4):337-41.

[11] Sodemann M, Jakobsen MS, Mølbak K, Alvarenga IC, Martins C, Aaby P. Malaria parasitemia and childhood diarrhea in a peri-urban area of Guinea-Bissau. *Am J Trop Med Hyg.* 1999 Aug;61(2):336-8.

[12] Luxemburger C, ter Kuile FO, Nosten F, Dolan G, Bradol JH, Phaipun L, Chongsuphajaisiddhi T, White NJ. Single day mefloquine-artesunate combination in the treatment of multi-drug resistant falciparum malaria. *Trans R Soc Trop Med Hyg.* 1994 Mar-Apr;88(2):213-7.

[13] ter Kuile FO, Nosten F, Luxemburger C, Kyle D, Teja-Isavatharm P, Phaipun L, Price R, Chongsuphajaisiddhi T, White NJ. Mefloquine treatment of acute falciparum malaria: a prospective study of non-serious adverse effects in 3673 patients. *Bull World Health Organ.* 1995;73(5):631-42.

[14] Bakshi R, Hermeling-Fritz I, Gathmann I, Alteri E. An integrated assessment of the clinical safety of artemether-lumefantrine: a new oral fixed-dose combination antimalarial drug. *Trans R Soc Trop Med Hyg.* 2000 Jul-Aug;94(4):419-24.

[15] Tjitra E, Suprianto S, Currie BJ, Morris PS, Saunders JR, Anstey NM. Therapy of uncomplicated falciparum malaria: a randomized trial comparing artesunate plus sulfadoxine-pyrimethamine versus sulfadoxine-pyrimethamine alone in Irian Jaya, Indonesia. *Am J Trop Med Hyg.* 2001 Oct;65(4):309-17.

[16] Ashley EA, McGready R, Hutagalung R, Phaiphun L, Slight T, Proux S, Thwai KL, Barends M, Looareesuwan S, White NJ, Nosten F. A randomized, controlled study of a simple, once-daily regimen of dihydroartemisinin-piperaquine for the treatment of

uncomplicated, multidrug-resistant falciparum malaria. *Clin Infect Dis*. 2005 Aug 15;41(4):425-32.

[17] Wattanakoon Y, Chittamas S, Pornkulprasit V, Kanda T, Thimasarn K, Rojanawatsirivej C, Looareesuwan S, Bunnag D. Six-years monitoring the efficacy of the combination of artesunate and mefloquine for the treatment of uncomplicated falciparum malaria. *Southeast Asian J Trop Med Public Health*. 2003 Sep;34(3):542-5.

[18] Coburn B, Grassl GA, Finlay BB. Salmonella, the host and disease: a brief review. *Immunol. Cell Biol*. 2007 Feb-Mar;85(2):112-8.

[19] Cooke FJ, Wain J. The emergence of antibiotic resistance in typhoid fever. *Travel. Med. Infect Dis*. 2004 Might;2(2):67-74.

[20] Su CP, Chen YC, Chang SC. Changing characteristics of typhoid fever in Taiwan. *J. Microbiol. Immunol. Infect*. 2004 Apr;37(2):109-14.

[21] Furuta I. Widal test. *Nippon Rinsho*. 2005 Jul;63 Suppl 7:142-5.

[22] Olopoenia LA, King AL. Widal agglutination test - 100 years later: still plagued by controversy. *Postgrad Med. J*. 2000 Feb;76(892):80-4.

[23] John TJ. Emerging & re-emerging bacterial pathogens in India. *Indian J Med Res*. 1996 Jan;103:4-18.

[24] Jog S, Soman R, Singhal T, Rodrigues C, Mehta A, Dastur FD. Enteric fever in Mumbai--clinical profile, sensitivity patterns and response to antimicrobials. *J Assoc Physicians India*. 2008 Apr;56:237-40.

[25] Patil AM, Kulkarni ML, Kulkarni AM. Baseline Widal titres in healthy children. *Indian J Pediatr*. 2007 Dec;74(12):1081-3.

[26] Dutta S, Sur D, Manna B, Sen B, Bhattacharya M, Bhattacharya SK, Wain J, Nair S, Clemens JD, Ochiai RL. Emergence of highly fluoroquinolone-resistant Salmonella enterica serovar Typhi in a community-based fever surveillance from Kolkata, India. *Int J Antimicrob Agents*. 2008 Apr;31(4):387-9.

[27] Palit A, Ghosh S, Dutta S, Sur D, Bhattacharya MK, Bhattacharya SK. Increasing prevalence of Salmonella enterica serotype Paratyphi-A in patients with enteric fever in a periurban slum setting of Kolkata, India. *Int J Environ Health Res*. 2006 Dec;16(6):455-9.

[28] Woods CW, Murdoch DR, Zimmerman MD, Glover WA, Basnyat B, Wolf L, Belbase RH, Reller LB. Emergence of Salmonella enterica serotype Paratyphi A as a major cause of enteric fever in Kathmandu, Nepal. *Trans R Soc Trop Med Hyg*. 2006 Nov;100(11):1063-7.

[29] Lakshmi V, Ashok R, Susmita J, Shailaja VV. Changing trends in the antibiograms of Salmonella isolates at a tertiary care hospital in Hyderabad. *Indian J Med Microbiol*. 2006 Jan;24(1):45-8.

[30] Mandal S, Mandal MD, Pal NK. Antibiotic resistance of Salmonella enterica serovar Paratyphi A in India: emerging and reemerging problem. *J Postgrad Med*. 2006 Jul-Sep;52(3):163-6.

[31] Manchanda V, Bhalla P, Sethi M, Sharma VK. Treatment of enteric fever in children on the basis of current trends of antimicrobial susceptibility of Salmonella enterica serovar typhi and paratyphi A. *Indian J Med Microbiol*. 2006 Apr;24(2):101-6.

[32] Fraser A, Goldberg E, Acosta CJ, Paul M, Leibovici L. Vaccines for preventing typhoid fever. *Cochrane Database Syst Rev*. 2007 Jul 18;(3):CD001261.

[33] Levine MM. Mass vaccination to control epidemic and endemic typhoid fever. *Curr Top Microbiol Immunol*. 2006;304:231-46.

[34] Panasiuk A. Vaccination for HIV positive travelers. *Przegl Epidemiol*. 2004;58 Suppl 1:97-100.

[35] Levine MM. Enteric infections and the vaccines to counter them: future directions. *Vaccine*. 2006 May 1;24(18):3865-73.

[36] Franklin QJ. Sudden death after typhoid and Japanese encephalitis vaccination in a young male taking pseudoephedrine. *Mil Med*. 1999 Feb;164(2):157-9.

[37] Cooper AL, Horan MA, Little RA, Rothwell NJ. Metabolic and febrile responses to typhoid vaccine in humans: effect of beta-adrenergic blockade. *J Appl Physiol*. 1992 Jun;72(6):2322-8.

[38] Cholera: assessing the risk to travellers and identifying means of prevention. *Travel Med. Infect. Dis*. 2003 Might;1(2):80-8.

[39] Fournier JM, Quilici ML. Cholera. Presse Med. 2007 Apr;36(4 Pt 2):727-39. *Epub*. 2007 Mar 1

[40] Cook CG. Gastroenterological emergencies in the tropics. *Baillieres Clin. Gastroenterol*. 1991 Dec;5(4):861-86.

[41] Saravanan V, Sanath Kumar H, Karunasagar I, Karunasagar I. Putative virulence genes of Vibrio cholerae from seafoods and the coastal environment of Southwest India. *Int J Food Microbiol*. 2007 Nov 1;119(3):329-33.

[42] Das S, Saha R, Kaur IR. Trend of antibiotic resistance of Vibrio cholerae strains from East Delhi. *Indian J Med Res*. 2008 May;127(5):478-82.

[43] Shukla I, Alam S. Emergence of Vibrio cholerae OI biotype EIT or serotype Inaba in Aligarh. *Indian J Pathol Microbiol*. 2007 Oct;50(4):938.

[44] Rajcshwari K, Gupta A, Dubey AP, Uppal B, Singh MM. Diarrhoeal outbreak of Vibrio cholerae 01 Inaba in Delhi. *Trop Doct*. 2008 Apr;38(2):105-7.

[45] Khuntia HK, Pal BB, Meher PK, Chhotray GP. Environmental Vibrio cholerae O139 may be the progenitor of outbreak of cholera in coastal area of Orissa, eastern India, 2000: molecular evidence. *Am J Trop Med Hyg*. 2008 May;78(5):819-22.

[46] Pal BB, Khuntia HK, Samal SK, Das SS, Chhotray GP. Emergence of Vibrio cholerae O1 biotype El Tor serotype Inaba causing outbreaks of cholera in Orissa, India. Jpn *J Infect Dis*. 2006 Aug;59(4):266-9.

[47] Roychowdhury A, Pan A, Dutta D, Mukhopadhyay AK, Ramamurthy T, Nandy RK, Bhattacharya SK, Bhattacharya MK. Emergence of tetracycline-resistant Vibrio cholerae O1 serotype Inaba, in Kolkata, *India. Jpn J Infect Dis*. 2008 Mar;61(2):128-9.

[48] Gupta DN, Mondal SK, Sarkar BL, Mukherjee S, Bhattacharya SK. An el tor cholera outbreak amongst tribal population in Tripura. *Commun Dis*. 2004 Dec;36(4):271-6.

[49] Taneja N, Biswal M, Tarai B, Sharma M. Emergence of Vibrio cholerae O1 Biotype El Tor serotype Inaba in north India. *Jpn J Infect Dis*. 2005 Aug;58(4):238-40.

[50] Gomber S, Mathur M, Sharma PP. Diarrhoeal outbreak of Vibrio cholerae 0139 from north India. *Acta Paediatr*. 1995 Feb;84(2):206-7.

[51] Griffith DC, Kelly-Hope LA, Miller MA. Review of reported cholera outbreaks worldwide, 1995-2005. *Am. J. Trop. Med. Hyg.* 2006 Nov;75(5):973-7.

[52] Taylor RK, Kirn TJ, Bose N, Stonehouse E, Tripathi SA, Kovác P, Wade WF. Progress towards development of a cholera subunit vaccine. *Chem. Biodivers.* 2004 Jul;1(7):1036-57.

[53] Chaignat CL. What about cholera vaccines? *Expert Rev Vaccines.* 2008 May;7(4):403-

[54] Olsson L, Parment PA. Present and future cholera vaccines. *Expert Rev Vaccines.* 2006 Dec;5(6):751-2.

[55] Lopez AL, Clemens JD, Deen J, Jodar L. Cholera vaccines for the developing world. *Hum Vaccin.* 2008 Mar-Apr;4(2):165-9.

[56] Graves P, Deeks J, Demicheli V, Pratt M, Jefferson T. Vaccines for preventing cholera. *Cochrane Database Syst Rev.* 2000;(4):CD000974.

[57] MacPherson DW, Tonkin M. Cholera vaccination: a decision analysis. *CMAJ.* 1992 Jun 1;146(11):1947-52.

[58] Nigoyi SK. Shigellosis. *J Microbiol.* 2005 Apr;43(2):133-43.

[59] Sur D, Ramamurthy T, Deen J, Bhattacharya SK. Shigellosis : challenges & management issues. *Indian J Med Res.* 2004 Nov;120(5):454-62.

[60] Bhattacharya SK. Progress in the prevention and control of diarrhoeal diseases since Independence. *Natl Med J India.* 2003;16 Suppl 2:15-9.

[61] Niyogi SK, Sarkar K, Lalmalsawma P, Pallai N, Bhattacharya SK. An outbreak of bacillary dysentery caused by quinolone-resistant Shigella dysenteriae type 1 in a northeastern state of India. *J Health Popul Nutr.* 2004 Mar;22(1):97.

[62] Singh J, Khanna KK, Sharma RS, Datta KK, Verghese T. An outbreak of shigellosis in a slum colony of Delhi-1990. *J Commun Dis.* 1993 Mar;25(1):41-2.

[63] Sengupta PG, Mandal S, Sen D, Das P, Deb BC, Pal SC.Multidrug resistant epidemic shigellosis in a village in west Bengal, 1984. *Indian J Public Health.* 1990 Jan-Mar;34(1):15-9.

[64] Datta P, Sen D. Outbreak of dysentery due to nalidixic acid resistant S. dysenteriae 1 at Agartala, Tripura: a hospital based study. *Indian J Public Health.* 1990 Jan-Mar;34(1):11-4.

[65] Virudhagini R. Poliovirus infection in the gastrointestinal tracts of children. *Indian Pediatr.* 2000 Feb;37(2):210-4.

[66] Nathanson N/ The pathogenesis of poliomyelitis: what we don't know. *Adv Virus Res.* 2008;71:1-50.

[67] Mandke VB, Pawar RM, Naik DD, Salgaonkar SD. An outbreak of poliomyelitis in the Marathwada region of Maharashtra State: 1990. Indian Pediatr. 1994 Sep;31(9):1091-4.

[68] Murthy N, Bhaskaram P, Murali MV, Sukanya M, Rao CR.An outbreak of poliomyelitis in Andhra Pradesh (South India). *Indian Pediatr.* 1994 May;31(5):533-41.

[69] Wadia NH, Katrak SM, Misra VP, Wadia PN, Miyamura K, Hashimoto K, Ogino T, Hikiji T, Kono R. Polio-like motor paralysis associated with acute hemorrhagic conjunctivitis in an outbreak in 1981 in Bombay, India: clinical and serologic studies. *J Infect Dis.* 1983 Apr;147(4):660-8.

[70] Lowalekar KB, Singh VD, Agrawal RL.Report on an epidemic of polio--like neuroparalytic disease associated with acute haemorrhagic conjunctivitis (A.H.C.). J Assoc Physicians India. 1983 Jun;31(6):339-42.

[71] Chakraborty S, Sehgal CL, Mathew KJ, George MJ. Poliomyelitis in Alleppey town, Kerala. J Commun Dis. 1984 Dec;16(4):328-9.

[72] Sundaravalli N, Narmada R, Sankar, Nedunchezian, Mukundan P. Spurt in poliomyelitis in Madras. Indian Pediatr. 1981 Aug;18(8):539-44.

[73] Saeed A, Kumar R, Srivastava AK, Rahman H, Agarwal VK. An outbreak of poliomyelitis in Allahabad. Indian Pediatr. 1980 Sep;17(9):757-61.

[74] Agarwal BL, Agarwal VK. Observations on a recent outbreak of poliomyelitis in Allahabad. J Indian Med Assoc. 1965 Dec 1;45(11):587-90.

[75] Paul Y. Polio eradication in India at the cross-roads. Vaccine. 2008 Sep 26. [Epub ahead of print]

[76] Phadke MA, Kshirsagar NA, Dalvi SD. Polio eradication for India: shift of focus. Vaccine. 2008 Aug 26;26(36):4625-6.

[77] Arya SC, Agarwal N. Polio eradication in India: the way forward. Indian J Pediatr. 200 Dec;74(12):1130.

Chapter IX

Emerging Hepatitis in India

Introduction to Tropical Hepatitis

Hepatitis by definition is the inflammation of the hepatic cell. There are many possible causes of hepatitis in medicine. These can be infectious or non-infectious. The hepatitis virus can be seen elsewhere around the world. However, high prevalence of hepatitis can be seen in the tropical regions. This might be due to the high rate of infectious hepatitis cases in this area. Concerning the signs and symptoms of hepatitis, the common presentation is jaundice, which implies disturbance of the bile system. Jaundice can be easily divided by its etiology as pre-hepatic, hepatic and post-hepatic types. However, jaundice does not mean injury or inflammation of hepatic cells. The direct reflection of the hepatic cell problem is the increased level of the hepatic enzyme. In laboratory medicine, the common liver function tests that imply the hepatic cellular condition are the two enzymes named SGOT and SGPT. These two enzymes are usually the basic diagnostic tools for hepatitis. The other hepatic profiles are not directly related to hepatic cellular disorder. Increased amounts of transaminase enzymes can be the clue for diagnosis of hepatitis. The other presentations of hepatitis include fever, fatigue, abdominal pain and myalgia, which are all weak signs and symptoms.

The term tropical hepatitis in this chapter means the condition of hepatitis that is specific to the nature of tropical countries. This can be either infection or non-infection related. Examples of infectious tropical hepatitis are several kinds of viral hepatitis diseases. Examples of non-infectious tropical hepatitis are several kinds of intoxications. When we talk about tropical hepatitis, ones usually tends to focus on the infection. Indeed, infection is a common problem in tropical countries and many infections can lead to the problem of hepatitis. The most common infectious disorder that brings tropical hepatitis is viral hepatitis. Viral hepatitis means the specific kind of hepatitis that is caused by the hepatitis virus. Hepatitis virus by definition means a group of viruses that can cause hepatitis in infected subjects. There are many kinds of hepatitis viruses that are still problematic around the world. There are several means of transmission. Details of each important hepatitis virus will be further discussed in this chapter.

Hepatitis A Virus Infection

Introduction [1 - 20]

The hepatitis A virus has been a well known virus in gastroenterology for a long time. This virus is transmitted via food contamination. The feco-oral route of transmission is mentioned.

The hepatitis A virus is a picornavirus. It is accepted as a common cause of hepatitis worldwide. Hepatitis A remains an important cause of community-acquired hepatitis in several countries especially for tropical, developing ones. Spread of infection is generally person to person or by oral intake after fecal contamination of skin or mucous membranes as already mentioned. In addition, there might be a scenario of fecal contamination of food or water. Hepatitis A is endemic in developing countries, and most residents are exposed in pediatric groups. Luckily, the adult population in developed countries demonstrates falling rates of exposure with improvements in hygiene and sanitation [1]. Presently, many tropical countries especially Asian countries are classified as endemic area for viral hepatitis A. In Asia, the hepatitis A infection is still an important viral infectious disease. A recent study indicated that almost all adults in developing countries in Asia had a natural immunity to this disease [2]. For years there have been reports on the outbreak of this infection in many countries. Concerning the reported outbreaks, there are both reports of the outbreak among the pediatric population and adult population. Usually, water is the main source of infection and untreated contaminated drinking water is often problematic [3 – 9]. Therefore, treated running tap water is important in prevention of hepatitis outbreaks, therefore, self -sanitation in drinking is very important in prevention. Recently, Wiwanitkit said that provision of clean water and control of possible contamination in drinking water as well as eating and drinking sanitation were the core concepts for hepatitis A prevention [10].

Table 1. Reports on the emergence of hepatitis A virus infection in India.

Authors	Details
Joshi et al [21]	Joshi et al reported on hepatitis A epidemic in Kerala state, India, in 1980 [21].
Skidmore et al [22]	Skidmore et al reported on an outbreak of hepatitis A on a hospital ward in India [22].
Sarguna et al [23]	Sarguna et al mentioned for diverse pattern of hepatitis A during the outbreak of hepatitis A in Hyderabad 2005 and made a question "is there a need for evolving newer strategies of vaccination? [23]"
Patnaik et al [24]	Patnaik et al reported on an outbreak of viral hepatitis A in Ibrahimpatnam town of Andhra Pradesh, India.

Hepatitis A Virus Infection in India

As previously noted, the hepatitis A virus infection can be classified as an important gastrointestinal infection. India is a country facing the problem of many gastrointestinal infections (more details in another specific chapter of this book). Hepatitis A virus infection in India is considered problematic. There are many reports on hepatitis A virus emerging in India. The summary of important reports is shown in Table 1.

Hepatitis B Virus Infection

Introduction [25 - 40]

Hepatitis B virus has been a well known virus in medicine for a long time. This virus is transmitted via blood and blood products. Also, it can be transmitted as a sexually transmitted disease. It is considered as a very important and highly contagious disease. The high rate of hepatitis B infection in Asia is considered a big public health problem. The difference from the hepatitis A infection, is that hepatitis B has a chronic form. The easy way to describe the fade of hepatitis B infection are the 5 C's: cure, carrier, chronic hepatitis, cirrhosis as well as carcinoma. The hepatocellular carcinoma is the totally unwanted outcome of hepatitis B infection. This is due to the process of chronic disturbance of liver cells by the virus. This is considered as a leading cause of death for many countries in tropical Asia. Hepatitis B is considered as a silent killer for millions of people. How to cope with the hepatitis B infection is of concern. Luckily, medical scientists succeeded in the production of hepatitis B vaccine. This vaccine is launched and helps control new cases of hepatitis B infection. It is recommended as an EPI vaccine for many countries in the endemic area. In addition, screening for hepatitis B virus is generally practiced. It is included in a set of screens for blood bank laboratories. In addition, there are also recommendations to screen for hepatitis B markers in many high-risk populations. The seromarker for hepatitis B virus is HBsAg. This is the basic investigation for diagnosis of disease. HBeAg is another important maker for making decisions on treatment of a HBsAg seropositive case. This marker is an indicator for the possibility of carcinogenesis. AntiHBc is the marker for a natural antibody. This means the antibody due to the previous infection of hepatitis B virus. AntiHBs is the marker for the response to the hepatitis B vaccination. It is detected in the vaccinees who respond to the vaccination.

Hepatitis B Virus Infection in India

As previously noted, hepatitis B virus infection can be classified as an important tropical infection. India is a country facing the problem of this specific viral infection. Hepatitis B virus infection in India is considered problematic and should be focused on. There are many reports on hepatitis B virus emerging in India. The summary of important reports is shown in Table 2.

Table 2. Reports on emerging hepatitis B virus infections in India.

Authors	Details
Singh et al [41]	Singh et al studied on a severe and explosive outbreak of hepatitis B in a rural population in Sirsa district, Haryana, India and reported that unnecessary therapeutic injections were a major risk factor [41].
Murhekar et al [42]	Murhekar et al noted for an alarming prevalence of hepatitis-B infection among the Jarawas, a primitive Negrito tribe of Andaman and Nicobar Islands, India [42].
Singh et al [43]	Singh et al reported on an outbreak of viral hepatitis B in a rural community in India linked to inadequately sterilized needles and syringes [43].
John et al [44]	John et al reported on epidemic hepatitis B caused by commercial human immunoglobulin in India [44].

Hepatitis C Virus Infection

Introduction [45 - 60]

Hepatitis C virus is a well known virus in medicine after the clarification of the so called non-A non-B viral hepatitis. This virus is transmitted via blood and blood products. Also, it can be transmitted as a sexually transmitted disease. It is considered a very important highly contagious disease. Although the prevalence of hepatitis C infection is not as high as that of hepatitis B infection in Asia it is still considered a big public health problem. The difference from hepatitis A infection but similar to hepatitis B, is that hepatitis C has a chronic form. The hepatocellular carcinoma is the totally unwanted outcome of hepatitis C infection. Similar to hepatitis B, this is due to the process of chronic disturbance of liver cells by the virus. Liver cancer is considered as a leading cause of death for many countries in tropical Asia. Hepatitis C is considered \ a silent killer for millions of people. How to cope with the hepatitis C infection is of concern. Unluckily, the medical scientists still have not succeeded in production of a hepatitis C vaccine. Screening for hepatitis B virus is not generally practiced. Screening for this virus is included in a set of screens for blood bank laboratories in some large settings.

Hepatitis C Virus Infection in India

As previously noted, hepatitis C virus infection can be classified as an important tropical infection. India is a country facing the problem of this specific viral infection. Hepatitis C virus infection in India is considered problematic and should be focused on. However, there is no report on emerging outbreaks of hepatitis C virus infection from India.

Hepatitis D Virus Infection

Introduction [61 - 75]

Hepatitis D virus is a well known virus in medicine after the clarification of its comparable nature to hepatitis B. This virus is transmitted via blood and blood products along with hepatitis B. Management of this hepatitis virus is not widely mentioned because of the nature of co-infection with hepatitis B. It is also managed the same way as for the hepatitis B virus infection.

Hepatitis D Virus Infection in India

As previously noted, the hepatitis D virus infection is not commonly mentioned as an important tropical infection. However, the hepatitis D virus infection in India is still concerning. Similar to hepatitis C, there is no report on emerging outbreaks of hepatitis D virus infection from India.

Hepatitis E Virus Infection

Introduction [76 - 95]

The hepatitis E virus has been a well known virus in gastroenterology for years. It is a non-enveloped, single-stranded, positive-sense RNA molecule of an approximately 7.2 kb length. This hepatitis virus is transmitted via food contamination. Feco-oral route of transmission is mentioned as main transmission means. It is accepted as another important food borne cause of hepatitis worldwide. Hepatitis E is still an important cause of community-acquired hepatitis in several countries especially for tropical developing countries in Asia. Spread of infection is generally person to person or by oral intake after fecal contamination of skin or by oral intake of contaminated food or water. Hepatitis E is endemic in developing countries and many tropical countries especially for Asian countries classified as endemic areas for viral hepatitis E, as already said. There have been reports on the emergence of this viral form of hepatitis in many countries for years. Concerning the reported outbreak, there are both reports of clusters among the pediatric population and adult population. Usually, water is the main source of infection and untreated contaminated drinking water must be focused on. Therefore, treated running tap water is important in prevention of hepatitis outbreak. Toilet, drinking and eating sanitation is very important in prevention. Recently, Wiwanitkit said that provision of clean water as well as eating and drinking sanitation were the major concepts for hepatitis A prevention [10] and this concept can be applied to hepatitis E because it shares the same means of transmission. It should also be noted that cases of acute hepatitis owing to novel HEV variants have been reported in humans without recognized risk factors for hepatitis E in Europe, Japan and the USA [95].

Hepatitis E Virus Infection in India

As previously mentioned, the hepatitis E virus infection can be accepted as an important gastrointestinal infection. India is a country facing the problem of many gastrointestinal infectious diseases (more details in another specific chapter of this book). The hepatitis E virus infection in India is considered problematic and should be focused on. There are many reports on the hepatitis E virus emerging in India. The summary of important reports is shown in Table 3.

Table 3. Reports on emerging hepatitis E virus infections in India.

Authors	Details
Sailaja et al [96]	Sailaja et al reported on outbreak of waterborne hepatitis E in Hyderabad, India, 2005 [96].
Sarguna et al [97]	Sarguna et al reported on outbreak of acute viral hepatitis due to hepatitis E virus in Hyderabad, India [97].
Ippagunta et al [98]	Ippagunta et al reported on presence of hepatitis E virus in sewage in Northern India focusing on its frequency and seasonal pattern [98].
Kumar et al [99]	Kumar et al reported on virological investigation of a hepatitis E epidemic in North India [99].
Arora et al [100]	Arora et al reported on hepatitis E infection in children from a study of an outbreak [100].
Arankalle et al [101]	Arankalle et al reported on the role of immune serum globulins in pregnant women during an epidemic of hepatitis E [101].
Neogi et al [102]	Neogi et al reported on an institutional outbreak of hepatitis E as a first time report from Calcutta city [102].
Singh et al [103]	Singh et al reported on an outbreak of viral hepatitis E focusing on role of community practices [103].
Naik et al [104]	Naik et al reported on a large waterborne viral hepatitis E epidemic in Kanpur, India [104].
Ray et al [105]	Ray et al reported on hepatitis E virus genome in stools of hepatitis patients during large epidemic in north India [105].

Hepatitis G Virus Infection

Introduction [106 - 114]

Hepatitis G virus has been a well known virus in medicine for a few years. This virus is transmitted via blood and blood products. The difference from other hepatitis virus infections and the nature of this infection is not well clarified. Whether hepatitis G infection induces cancer is of concern. Unluckily, medical scientists have still not succeeded in the production of a hepatitis G vaccine. Screening for hepatitis G virus is not generally practiced. Screening for this virus is also not included in a set of screens for blood bank laboratory practice.

Hepatitis G Virus Infection in India

As previously noted, the hepatitis G virus infection can be classified as an important tropical infection. India is a country facing the problem of this specific viral infection. Hepatitis G virus infection in India is considered problematic and should be focused on. However, there is no report on emerging outbreaks of hepatitis G virus infection from India.

References

[1] Cuthbert JA. Hepatitis A: old and new. *Clin Microbiol Rev* 2001;14:38-58.

[2] Burke DS, Snitbhan R, Johnson DE, Scott RM. Age-specific prevalence of hepatitis A virus antibody in Thailand. *Am J Epidemiol* 1981;113:245-9.

[3] Pathanapornpandh N, Paisalsilp S, Patchakkhapat K. Hepatitis A outbreak in a primary school, Suratthani. *Commun Dis J* 1986; 12: 360-378.

[4] Watanasi S, Oonhalekhaka A, Kaewnokkhao W, Khongket K, Chatsanga C, Toraksa K,Suriyamongkhon W.An epidemic of viral hepatitis A in the Police Cadet Academy. *Thai Pol Med J* 1987; 13: 205-222.

[5] Phonboon K, Kasitipradit N, Lilapongse W, Paopradit M, Mobnarin S, Lailang W, Buchakorn L, Raksapol S, Sukkua T. Hepatitis outbreak due to municipal piped water in Tungsong, Nakhon Si Thammarat. *Commun Dis J* 1984; 10: 14-36.

[6] Siriarayaporn P, Sae-jeng K, Phunawakul U, Chittrapitaklerd S, Chuthasmith K, Peerapattanapokin V, Pokhawattana L, Wannasilp K, Khonthong P, Wangsrisiripeth S, Phurahong S, Kerdkhai S, Boonmardee A. A report on epidemiology surveillance of hepatitis A epidemic in a factory in Yannawa district, Bangkok. *Month Epidemiol Surveil Rep* 1994;3: 693-96, 703-705.

[7] Phunawakool U, Warintharawart S, Sanitpunt R, Chaikhun W. Outbreak of hepatitis A in Saraburi Province, October 1992. *W Epidemiol Surveil* Rep 1993; 24: 621-2 , 629-313.8.

[8] Rungsin R, Punnachet K, Peerapattanapokin V, Chitpitaklerd S, Siriarayaporn P,Thammapornpilard P, Khonthong P, Phurahong S, Wangsrisiripeth S, Naruphonchirakul U, Argkhean N, Khumnurak U, Kongsiri K. Results from epidemiology surveillance of hepatitis A epidemic in "Soongsumarnwit" Bangparma school during 2 – 3 September, 1993. *W Epidemiol Surveil* Rep 1995; 26 : 373-376, 383-387.

[9] Appleton H. Control of food-borne viruses. *Br Med Bull* 2000;56:172-83.

[10] Wiwanitkit V. Hepatitis A outbreak in Thailand during the past 25-year period, a summary. *Rev Esp Enferm Dig*. 2008 Feb;100(2):115-6.

[11] Shulman NR, Hirschman RJ, Barker LF. Viral hepatitis. *Ann Intern Med.* 1970 Feb;72(2):257-69.

[12] Krejs GJ, Gassner M, Blum AL. Epidemiology of infectious hepatitis. *Clin Gastroenterol.* 1974 May;3(2):277-303.

[13] Waterson AP. The viruses of hepatitis. Clin Gastroenterol. 1974 May;3(2):241-54.

[14] Kaboth U, Junge U. Prophylaxis of viral hepatitis. *Clin Gastroenterol.* 1974 May;3(2):453-70.

[15] Nikonova TN. Viral hepatitis in children. *Pediatriia.* 1974;53(5):77-81.

[16] Krugman S. Hepatitis virus vaccines: present status. *Yale J Biol Med.* 1982 May-Aug;55(3-4):375-81.

[17] Zhkarinsky E, Rubin E. The biology of viral hepatitis. *Monogr Pathol.* 1982;(23):156-87.

[18] Lund E. Waterborne virus diseases. *Ecol Dis.* 1982;1(1):27-35.

[19] Tkacheva MN, Lobanova EA, Atkian RV. Viral hepatitis--a world health problem. *Zh Mikrobiol Epidemiol Immunobiol.* 1981 Sep;(9):6-13.

[20] Skinhøj P. Epidemiological aspects of viral hepatitis A and B infections. A review with special reference to serological studies in isolated areas. *Dan Med Bull.* 1981 Oct;28(5):177-92.

[21] Joshi YK, Tandon BN, Gandhi BM. Hepatitis A epidemic in Kerala state (India) in 1980. *Indian J Med Res.* 1985 Jan;81:96-101

[22] Skidmore SJ, Gully PR, Middleton JD, Hassam ZA, Singal GM. An outbreak of hepatitis A on a hospital ward. *J Med Virol.* 1985 Oct;17(2):175-7.

[23] Sarguna P, Rao A, Ramana KN. Diverse pattern of hepatitis A during the outbreak of AVH in Hyderabad 2005: is there a need for evolving newer strategies of vaccination? *Indian J Pathol Microbiol.* 2007 Oct;50(4):939-40.

[24] Patnaik SK, Bandyopadhyay S, Sharma RS, Datta KK. An outbreak of viral hepatitis A in Ibrahimpatnam town of Andhra Pradesh. *J Commun Dis.* 1995 Jun;27(2):118-9.

[25] Rantala M, van de Laar MJ.Surveillance and epidemiology of hepatitis B and C in Europe - a review. *Euro Surveill.* 2008 May 22;13(21). pii: 18880.

[26] Lindh M, Uhnoo I, Bläckberg J, Duberg AS, Friman S, Fischler B, Karlström O, Norkrans G, Reichard O, Sangfeldt P, Söderström A, Sönnerborg A, Weiland O, Wejstål R, Wiström J Treatment of chronic hepatitis B infection: an update of Swedish recommendations. *Scand J Infect Dis.* 2008;40(6-7):436-8.

[27] Yoon SK.Recent advances in tumor markers of human hepatocellular carcinoma. *Intervirology.* 2008;51 Suppl 1:34-41

[28] Sakamoto M, Mori T, Masugi Y, Effendi K, Rie I, Du W. Candidate molecular markers for histological diagnosis of early hepatocellular carcinoma. *Intervirology.* 2008;51 Suppl 1:42-5.

[29] La Vecchia C. Cancer and liver cancer prevention: is it a fact or just a potential? *Hepatology.* 2008 Jul;48(1):7-9.

[30] McMahon BJ. Natural history of chronic hepatitis B - clinical implications. *Medscape J Med.* 2008 Apr 16;10(4):91.

[31] Van Bambeke F. The ABC of viral hepatitis. *J Pharm Belg.* 2008 Mar;63(1):15-20.

[32] Cheung YS, Chan HL, Wong J, Lee KF, Poon TC, Wong N, Lai PB. Elevated perioperative transaminase level predicts intrahepatic recurrence in hepatitis B-related hepatocellular carcinoma after curative hepatectomy. *Asian J Surg*. 2008 Apr;31(2):41-9.

[33] Kumada H. Advance in technical method and treatment for viral hepatitis. Rinsho Byori. 2008 Feb;56(2):108-13.

[34] Loomba R, Rowley A, Wesley R, Liang TJ, Hoofnagle JH, Pucino F, Csako G. Systematic review: the effect of preventive lamivudine on hepatitis B reactivation during chemotherapy. *Ann Intern Med.* 2008 Apr 1;148(7):519-28.

[35] Dayaram T, Marriott SJ. Effect of transforming viruses on molecular mechanisms associated with cancer. *J Cell Physiol.* 2008 Aug;216(2):309-14

[36] Honda M, Kaneko S. Sustained hepatitis virus infection and development of liver cancer. 1. Hepatic carcinogenesis associated with viral hepatitis. Nippon Naika Gakkai Zasshi. 2008 Jan 10;97(1):82-91

[37] Aikata H, Chayama K. Practice of screening tests for a group of patients with a high risk of developing liver cancer. Nippon Naika Gakkai Zasshi. 2008 Jan 10;97(1):23-7

[38] But DY, Lai CL, Yuen MF.Natural history of hepatitis-related hepatocellular carcinoma. *World J Gastroenterol.* 2008 Mar 21;14(11):1652-6

[39] Hagymási K, Tulassay Z. Epidemiology, risk factors and molecular pathogenesis of primary liver cancer. *Orv Hetil.* 2008 Mar 23;149(12):541-8

[40] Hann HW. Active antiviral therapy for chronic hepatitis B and hepatocellular carcinoma. *Minerva Gastroenterol Dietol.* 2008 Mar;54(1):19-30.

[41] Singh J, Gupta S, Khare S, Bhatia R, Jain DC, Sokhey J. A severe and explosive outbreak of hepatitis B in a rural population in Sirsa district, Haryana, India: unnecessary therapeutic injections were a major risk factor. *Epidemiol Infect.* 2000 Dec;125(3):693-9.

[42] Murhekar MV, Murhekar KM, Sehgal SC. Alarming prevalence of hepatitis-B infection among the Jarawas--a primitive Negrito tribe of Andaman and Nicobar Islands, India. *J Viral Hepat.* 2003 May;10(3):232-3.

[43] Singh J, Bhatia R, Gandhi JC, Kaswekar AP, Khare S, Patel SB, Oza VB, Jain DC, Sokhey J. Outbreak of viral hepatitis B in a rural community in India linked to inadequately sterilized needles and syringes. *Bull World Health Organ.* 1998;76(1):93-8.

[44] John TJ, Ninan GT, Rajagopalan MS, John F, Flewett TH, Francis DP, Zuckerman AJ. Epidemic hepatitis B caused by commercial human immunoglobulin. *Lancet.* 1979 May 19;1(8125):1074.

[45] Balsano C, Alisi A. Hepatitis C virus (HCV): an RNA virus with a pro-oncogenic potential. *Dig Liver Dis*. 2007 Sep;39 Suppl 1:S46-51

[46] Abbasoglu O. Liver transplantation: yesterday, today and tomorrow. World *J Gastroenterol.* 2008 May 28;14(20):3117-22

[47] Acharya JN, Pacheco VH.Neurologic complications of hepatitis C. *Neurologist*. 2008 May;14(3):151-6.

[48] Foster G, Mathurin P.Hepatitis C virus therapy to date. *Antivir Ther*. 2008;13 Suppl 1:3-8.

[49] Willatt JM, Hussain HK, Adusumilli S, Marrero JA. MR Imaging of hepatocellular carcinoma in the cirrhotic liver: challenges and controversies. *Radiology.* 2008 May;247(2):311-30

[50] Hoofnagle JH, Seeff LB. Peginterferon and ribavirin for chronic hepatitis C. *N Engl J Med.* 2006 Dec 7;355(23):2444-51

[51] Moradpour D, Blum HE. Therapy of hepatitis C. *Praxis* (Bern 1994). 2002 May 29;91(22):977-82.

[52] Pawlotsky JM. Therapy of hepatitis C: from empiricism to eradication. *Hepatology.* 2006 Feb;43(2 Suppl 1):S207-20.

[53] Zeuzem S. Combination therapy for chronic viral hepatitis C. Dtsch Med Wochenschr. 2003 Feb 21;128(8):370-4.

[54] Niederau C, Kaden T. Therapy of chronic Hepatitis C in 2008. MMW Fortschr Med. 2008 Mar 27;150(13):31-4.

[55] Santantonio T, Wiegand J, Tilman Gerlach J. Acute hepatitis C: Current status and remaining challenges. *J Hepatol.* 2008 Oct;49(4):625-33.

[56] Maheshwari A, Ray S, Thuluvath PJ. Acute hepatitis C. *Lancet.* 2008 Jul 26;372(9635):321-32.

[57] Szabo G, Dolganiuc A. Hepatitis C and innate immunity: recent advances. *Clin Liver Dis.* 2008 Aug;12(3):675-92, x.

[58] Kotlyar DS, Blonski W, Rustgi VK. Noninvasive monitoring of hepatitis C fibrosis progression. *Clin Liver Dis.* 2008 Aug;12(3):557-71, viii.

[59] Paik SW. Goals of treatment, indication, and treatment for chronic hepatitis C. *Korean J Gastroenterol.* 2008 Jun;51(6):368-71.

[60] Shiffman ML. Optimizing the current therapy for chronic hepatitis C virus: peginterferon and ribavirin dosing and the utility of growth factors. *Clin Liver Dis.* 2008 Aug;12(3):487-505, vii.

[61] Husa P, Linhartová A, Nemecek V, Husová L. Hepatitis D. *Acta Virol.* 2005;49(4):219-25.

[62] Inoue O, Nakagawa Y, Mawatari H. Diagnostic tests: Hepatitis delta virus (HDV) marker. *Nippon Rinsho.* 2005 Jul;63 Suppl 7:418-20.

[63] Suda T, Ohkoshi S, Aoyagi Y. Detection of HDV-RNA. *Nippon Rinsho.* 2004 Aug;62 Suppl 8:416-9.

[64] Ogata N. Hepatitis delta (D) virus infection: general aspects of epidemiology, infection modes and clinical picture. *Nippon Rinsho.* 2004 Aug;62 Suppl 8:406-11.

[65] Inoue O, Nakagawa Y, Mawatari H. Detection of HDV antigen and antibody. *Nippon Rinsho.* 2004 Aug;62 Suppl 8:412-5.

[66] Farci P. Delta hepatitis: an update. J Hepatol. 2003;39 Suppl 1:S212-9.

[67] Ohishi W, Chayama K. Hepatitis D virus infection. *Nippon Rinsho.* 2003 Feb;61 Suppl 2:245-8.

[68] Ogata N. Hepatitis delta (D) virus genome: unique structure and replication, and their implication in the pathogenicity. *Nippon Rinsho.* 2003 Mar;61 Suppl 3:634-9.

[69] Fonseca JC. Hepatitis D. *Rev Soc Bras Med Trop.* 2002 Mar-Apr;35(2):181-90.

[70] Bean P. Latest discoveries on the infection and coinfection with hepatitis D virus. *Am Clin Lab.* 2002 Jun;21(5):25-7.

[71] Fabrizi F, Lunghi G, Martin P. Epidemiology of hepatitis delta virus (HDV) infection in the dialysis population. *Int J Artif Organs*. 2002 Jan;25(1):8-17.

[72] Abiad H, Ramani R, Currie JB, Hershow RC. The natural history of hepatitis D virus infection in Illinois state facilities for the developmentally disabled. *Am J Gastroenterol.* 2001 Feb;96(2):534-40.

[73] Rizzetto M. Hepatitis D: virology, clinical and epidemiological aspects. *Acta Gastroenterol Belg*. 2000 Apr-Jun;63(2):221-4.

[74] Inoue O, Yano M. Delta hepatitis virus (HDV) marker. *Nippon Rinsho*. 1999 Nov;57 Suppl:356-8.

[75] Arase Y, Kumada H. Hepatitis D. Ryoikibetsu Shokogun Shirizu. 1999;(23 Pt 1):59-61.

[76] Haagsma EB, van den Berg AP, Porte RJ, Benne CA, Vennema H, Reimerink JH, Koopmans MP. Chronic hepatitis E virus infection in liver transplant recipients. *Liver Transpl*. 2008 Apr;14(4):547-53.

[77] Mushahwar IK. Hepatitis E virus: molecular virology, clinical features, diagnosis, transmission, epidemiology, and prevention. *J Med Virol*. 2008 Apr;80(4):646-58.

[78] Purcell RH, Emerson SU. Hepatitis E: an emerging awareness of an old disease. *J Hepatol*. 2008 Mar;48(3):494-503.

[79] Kato T, Takahashi K. Attention-getting zoonoses: *Hepatitis E*. Nippon Naika Gakkai Zasshi. 2007 Nov 10;96(11):2418-22.

[80] Emerson SU, Purcell RH. *Hepatitis E. Pediatr Infect Dis J*. 2007 Dec;26(12):1147-8.

[81] Jiménez de Oya N, Escribano-Romero E, Blázquez AB, Saiz JC. Hepatitis E virus: zoonotic implications. *Gastroenterol Hepatol*. 2007 Aug-Sep;30(7):408-18.

[82] Dalton HR, Fellows HJ, Stableforth W, Joseph M, Thurairajah PH, Warshow U, Hazeldine S, Remnarace R, Ijaz S, Hussaini SH, Bendall RP. The role of hepatitis E virus testing in drug-induced liver injury. *Aliment Pharmacol Ther.* 2007 Nov 15;26(10):1429-35.

[83] Panda SK, Thakral D, Rehman S. Hepatitis E virus. *Rev Med Virol*. 2007 May-Jun;17(3):151-80.

[84] Teo CG. Hepatitis E indigenous to economically developed countries: to what extent a zoonosis? *Curr Opin Infect Dis*. 2006 Oct;19(5):460-6.

[85] Okamoto H. Hepatitis E. Nippon Naika Gakkai Zasshi. 2006 May 10;95(5):945-51.

[86] Bäcklund P, Raahenmaa M. Hepatitis E infections as a world wide problem] *Duodecim*. 2005;121(22):2443-7.

[87] Tanaka E. Diagnostic tests: Hepatitis E viral marker. *Nippon Rinsho*. 2005 Jul;63 Suppl 7:421-3.

[88] Mikhaĭlov MI, Zamiatina NA, Poleshchuk VF. Viral hepatitis E. The problems of its study. *Vopr Virusol*. 2005 May-Jun;50(3):20-2.

[89] Goens SD, Perdue ML. Hepatitis E viruses in humans and animals. *Anim Health Res Rev*. 2004 Dec;5(2):145-56.

[90] Nikami T, Hijikata M, Masaki N, Hayashi S. Detection of HEV-RNA. *Nippon Rinsho*. 2004 Aug;62 Suppl 8:546-7.

[91] Takeda N, Li TC, Miyamura T. Detection of antibodies of HEV. *Nippon Rinsho*. 2004 Aug;62 Suppl 8:542-5.

[92] Tanaka E. Outline of hepatitis E. Nippon Rinsho. 2004 Aug;62 Suppl 8:536-41.

[93] Takeda N, Li TC, Miyamura T. Structure of HEV. *Nippon Rinsho.* 2004 Aug;62 Suppl 8:501-3.

[94] Pérez-Gracia MT, Rodríguez-Iglesias M. Hepatitis E virus: current status. *Med Clin* (Barc). 2003 Dec 6;121(20):787-92.

[95] Sailaja B, Murhekar MV, Hutin YJ, Kuruva S, Murthy SP, Reddy KS, Rao GM, Gupte MD. Outbreak of waterborne hepatitis E in Hyderabad, India, 2005. *Epidemiol Infect.* 2008 Jul 7:1-7. [Epub ahead of print]

[96] Sarguna P, Rao A, Sudha Ramana KN. Outbreak of acute viral hepatitis due to hepatitis E virus in Hyderabad. *Indian J Med Microbiol.* 2007 Oct;25(4):378-82.

[97] Ippagunta SK, Naik S, Sharma B, Aggarwal R. Presence of hepatitis E virus in sewage in Northern India: frequency and seasonal pattern. *J Med Virol.* 2007 Dec;79(12):1827-31.

[98] Kumar S, Ratho RK, Chawla YK, Chakraborti A.Virological investigation of a hepatitis E epidemic in North India. *Singapore Med J.* 2006 Sep;47(9):769-73.

[99] Arora NK, Panda SK, Nanda SK, Ansari IH, Joshi S, Dixit R, Bathla R. Hepatitis E infection in children: study of an outbreak. *J Gastroenterol Hepatol.* 1999 Jun;14(6):572-7.

[100] Arankalle VA, Chadha MS, Dama BM, Tsarev SA, Purcell RH, Banerjee K. Role of immune serum globulins in pregnant women during an epidemic of hepatitis E. *J Viral Hepat.* 1998 May;5(3):199-204.

[101] Neogi DK, Bhattacharya N, De PN, Chakravarti T, Hati AK, Prakash C, Datta KK, Mukherjee KK. An institutional outbreak of hepatitis E--reported first time from Calcutta city. *J Commun Dis.* 1995 Dec;27(4):229-33.

[102] Singh J, Aggarwal NR, Bhattacharjee J, Prakash C, Bora D, Jain DC, Sharma RS, Datta KK. An outbreak of viral hepatitis E: role of community practices. *J Commun Dis.* 1995 Jun;27(2):92-6.

[103] Naik SR, Aggarwal R, Salunke PN, Mehrotra NN. A large waterborne viral hepatitis E epidemic in Kanpur, India. *Bull World Health Organ.* 1992;70(5):597-604.

[104] Ray R, Aggarwal R, Salunke PN, Mehrotra NN, Talwar GP, Naik SR. Hepatitis E virus genome in stools of hepatitis patients during large epidemic in north India. *Lancet.* 1991 Sep 28;338(8770):783-4.

[105] Sehgal R, Sharma A. Hepatitis G virus (HGV): current perspectives. *Indian J Pathol Microbiol.* 2002 Jan;45(1):123-8.

[106] Kleinman S. Hepatitis G virus biology, epidemiology, and clinical manifestations: Implications for blood safety. *Transfus Med Rev.* 2001 Jul;15(3):201-12.

[107] Kiyosawa K, Tanaka E. GB virus C/Hepatitis G virus. *Intervirology.* 1999;42(2-3):185-95.

[108] Heinsen A, Fomsgaard A. Hepatitis G virus or hepatitis GB virus C. Ugeskr Laeger. 1999 May 3;161(18):2653-6

[109] Sarrazin C, Roth WK, Zeuzem S. GB virus-C/hepatitis G virus--discovery, epidemiology, diagnosis and clinical relevance. *Z Gastroenterol.* 1998 Nov;36(11):997-1008.

[110] Rambusch EG, Wedemeyer H, Tillmann HL, Heringlake S, Manns MP. Significance of coinfection with hepatitis G virus for chronic hepatitis C--a review of the literature. *Z Gastroenterol.* 1998 Jan;36(1):41-53

[111] Poovorawan Y, Theamboonlers A, Hirsch P. Does hepatitis G virus cause significant clinical liver disease? *Southeast Asian J Trop Med Public Health.* 1997 Dec;28(4):678-82.

[112] Berenguer M, Berenguer J. Hepatitis G virus (HGV). *Gastroenterol Hepatol.* 1996 Dec;19(10):529-33.

[113] Tanaka E. GB virus C/hepatitis G virus infection in patients with chronic non-B, non-C hepatitis. *Nippon Rinsho.* 1997 Mar;55(3):559-63.

Chapter X

Tuberculosis in India

Introduction [1 - 30]

Tuberculosis is one of the most important infectious diseases in the world. On average, one-third of the world's population is expected to get this infection. There are millions of people who get new infections annually. There are also millions of deaths due to tuberculosis every year. The diagnosis and treatment of tuberculosis are known by physicians around the world. The common clinical presentation of tuberculosis include the chronic cough (for more than 3 months), hemoptysis, low grade fever, fatigue, night sweating, as well as weight loss. However, these symptoms are not specific. There are also many other tropical infections that can provide similar symptoms.

The etiological pathogen for tuberculosis is a bacteria named *Mycobacterium tuberculosis*. It is classified as acid fast bacillus (AFB), which can be stained in red due to AFB staining. It can be detected in the lung of infected, untreated patients. The patients usually get the pathogen from infected cases via an infected aerosphere in the contaminated atmosphere. The pathogen can be free in air for a week. Concerning the sputum, the pathogen can be persistent for half a year. The spreading of the pathogen is mainly via the respirator tract. There are also reports of other modes of transmission including mother to child via placenta. Basically, this disease is common in the poor due to poor sanitation. The patients can be symptomless and the chest X-ray might not reveal a lung lesion. The tuberculin can be useful. Due to the arising of HIV infection, the TB infection emerges. The atypical TB infection becomes a new problem among the HIV infected cases.

The period of time from getting the germ to a positive tuberculin result is about 2 – 10 weeks. In case the host is healthy, infection cannot occur. However, as already said, poor immune conditions will cause flaring of the disease. Although BCG prevention is globally recommended, the immune impairment due to HIV infection is the major factor causing the remergence of TB around the world. Mainly, TB infection usually manifests as a respiratory tract infection. Main respiratory presentations include chronic cough and hemoptysis. Some cases may present chest pain, especially in the case of pleuritis complication. Extrapulmonary TB infection can be seen but is less common. The important extrapulmonary manifestations include TB lymphadenopathy and TB meningitis. TB lymphadenopathy will present as an unexplained enlargement of lymph nodes. Some cases may have ruptures in the sinus tract and could also cause ulcers. Concerning the TB meningitis, the patients may have chronic fever as well as meningeal signs. Cerebrospinal fluid examination can be helpful.

Concerning the diagnosis of TB, the chest X ray is routinely used. From the chest X ray, abnormal lung lesion can be seen. However, its specificity is low, therefore, additional tests should be used. Sputum examination and AFB staining are usually indicated. This technique is highly specific but has low sensitivity. The staining technique is easy and fast to do. Considering sputum culture, it takes a long time and has complicated processes therefore it is not routinely used. For classification of TB, it is routinely based on sputum AFB result. Two main groups are classified. The first group is called smear positive group. This is the case that has positive sputum AFB examination with abnormal chest X-ray or a case that has two times the positive sputum examination without a chest X-ray. The second group is called smear negative group. This is the case that has negative sputum AFB examination but positive chest X=ray or a case that has negative sputum AFB result with positive sputum culture.

For treatment, standard regimen for TB treatment (2HRZE + 4HR) is widely used. However, the problem of drug resistance is emerging and becomes the problem in present medicine. Considering treatment of TB, the favorable results can be expected if correct regimen is used and the patient regularly takes the antituberculous drug for the complete course as per recommendation. If there is a failure, the possible causes include a) the patient does not regularly take the antituberculous drug for complete course as per recommendation, b) physician does not select correct regimen, c) a drug allergy existed, d) drug resistance occurs and e) the patient has impaired immune status (such as in HIV infected cases).

Table 1. Standard antituberculos drug.

drugs	dosage
Isoniazid (H)	10 mg/kg
Rifampicin (R)	10 mg/kg
Pyrazinamide (Z)	35 mg/kg
Ethambutol (E)	30 mg/kg

*The main adverse effects due to antituberculous drug taking are hepatitis and dermatitis. If these adverse effects occur, stopping of all drugs are recommended.

** Pyrazinamide is contraindicated in pregnancy.

"LIPF", is it Specific in Human Pathogenic Mycobacterium ?

1. Introduction

Over recent years, tuberculosis (TB) and disease caused by the human immunodeficiency virus (HIV) have merged in a new fashion of synergistic pandemic [31]. In many countries, where HIV is driving an emergence of the TB burden, the capacity of the current tools and strategies to reduce the burden has been exceeded [1]. The presence of cachectin or tumor necrosis factor (TNF) related to hypertriglyceridemia was demonstrated in the serum of patients with pulmonary tuberculosis [32]. The hyperlipidemia that accompanies this infection might be modified by the TNF inhibition of lipoprotein lipase activity [32]. This sequence of events can be sufficient to explain, in part, the complex metabolic changes and emaciation seen in tuberculosis patients [32]. Putative lipase, Rv3487c (lipF), a member of the lipase family of *Mycobacterium tuberculosis*, is strongly related to the virulence of the tuberculous pathogen [33]. This enzyme can be used for differentiation between different species of Mycobacterium [34]. To study the function of LIPF in different species of Mycobacterium, the new development in bioinformatics can be applied. Here, the author used a new gene ontology technology to predict the molecular function of LIPF from different species of Mycobacterium.

2. Materials and Methods

2.1. Finding the Sequence

The database PubMed was used for data mining of the amino acid sequence for LIPF of Mycobacterium species.

2.2. Prediction of Molecular Function and Biological Process

The author performs predictions of molecular functions and biological processes of normal and each abnormal hemoglobin using a novel gene ontology prediction tool, GoFigure [35]. GoFigure is a computational tool which was recently developed in gene ontology [35]. The prediction of molecular function were presented and compared.

3. Results

3.1. Sequence of LIPF in Different Mycobacterium Species

From searching the database of LIPF, sequence of *M. bovis* AF2122/97 and *M. tuberculosis* H37Rv can be derived and used for further study.

3.2. Prediction of Molecular Function and Biological Process

Using GoFigure server, the molecular function in *M. bovis* AF2122/97 and *M. tuberculosis* H37Rv is predicted. The molecular functions of LIPF of both species are similar as presented in Figure 1.

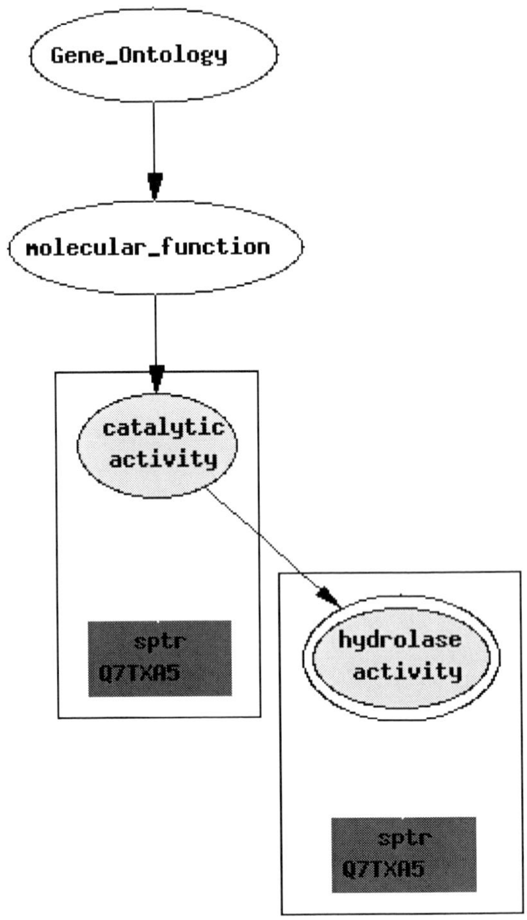

Figure 1. Predicted molecular function of LIPF in *M. bovis* AF2122/97 and *M. tuberculosis* H37Rv.

4. Discussion

New developments have forced a re-evaluation of our understanding of the structure and function of the Mycobacterium enzyme. Lipase is an enzyme, which is necessary for Mycobacterium. The presence of lipase, in Mycobacterium species gotten from tissues, has been detected by showing the ability of the bacteria to hydrolyze tributyrin [36]. LIPF is an important enzyme that is proposed to relate to the pathogenesis of disease in humans [33]. Failure of phagosomes containing *M. tuberculosis* to acidify is noted to relate to LIPF [37]. Until recently, the function of LIPF in different Mycobacterium species had not been well explored and there is a need for better understanding on those proteins' functions.

Compared to *M. tuberculosis, the M. bovis* has the same function. Of interest, the function in human pathogenic and non-pathogenic species is the same. It has been mentioned that the LIPF is not a species specific virulent factor. However, further experimental studies are needed before reaching a conclusion on this topic. The findings in this study not only support the previous knowledge on bacterial enzyme but also give a new view on the function of pathogenesis.

Tuberculosis in India

1. General Concern

India is a big country. There are also some areas facing the problem of emerging tuberculosis. Indeed, tuberculosis can be classified as an important re-emerging infection in India. There are many reports on the emergence of tuberculosis in India as shown in Table 2.

Table 2. Reports on the emergence of tuberculosis in India.

Author	Details
Williams et al [38]	Williams et al reported on the impact of HIV/AIDS on the control of tuberculosis in India [38].
Murali and Sajjan [39]	Murali and Sajjan discussed DOTS strategy for control of tuberculosis epidemic [39].
Karande and Bavdekar [40]	Karande and Bavdekar reported on multidrug-resistant tuberculosis in Mumbai (Bombay), India [40].
Balasubramanian et al [41]	Balasubramanian et al reported direct observation of anti-tuberculosis treatment and patient outcomes, Kerala State, India [41].
Sawert [42]	Sawert implied re-emergence of tuberculosis and its economic implications [42].

2. Multidrug Resistant Tuberculosis

Multidrug resistant tuberculosis is the tuberculosis that is resistant to at least both isoniazia and rifampicin. This condition has contributed to the problematic TB infectious cases. Multiple drug resistant tuberculosis is emerging as one of the most problematic infectious diseases in medical history. It is thought to have been created by medical personnel who administered anti-TB drugs improperly. The required time for treatment is longer than in normal conditions. The sputum culture and sensitivity test is indicated by a following up of treatment. Long term treatment (2 – 3 years) with close follow-ups is needed and the parenteral antituberculous drug is usually required. This problem is also observed in India and presently, is still a problem. Some important reports are presented in Table 3.

Table 3. Reports on multidrug resistant tuberculosis in India.

Author	Details
Mondal and Jain [43]	Mondal and Jain mentioned an extensively drug-resistant *Mycobacterium tuberculosis*, India [43].
Karande and Bavdekar [40]	Karande and Bavdekar reported on pediatric patients with multidrug-resistant tuberculosis in Mumbai (Bombay), India [40].
Almeida et al [44]	Almeida et al mentioned a high incidence of the Beijing genotype among multidrug-resistant isolates of *Mycobacterium tuberculosis* in a tertiary care center in Mumbai, India [44].
Suresh et al [45]	Suresh et al reported on rpoB gene sequencing and spoligotyping of multidrug-resistant *Mycobacterium tuberculosis* isolates from India [45].
Singh et al [46]	Singh et al reported on high rate of extensively drug-resistant tuberculosis in Indian AIDS patients [46].
Mistry et al [47]	Mistry et al reported on spoligotyping of Mycobacterium tuberculosis isolates from multiple-drug-resistant tuberculosis patients from Bombay, India [47].
Almeida et al [48]	Almeida et al reported on incidence of multidrug-resistant tuberculosis in urban and rural India and implications for prevention [48].
Harris et al [49]	Harris et al reported on genetic diversity and evidence for acquired antimicrobial resistance in Mycobacterium tuberculosis at a large hospital in South India [49].
Mahajan et al [50]	Mahajan et al reported on initial and acquired drug resistance of Mycobacterium tuberculosis in east Delhi, India [50]
Sulochana et al [51]	Sulochana et al reported on analysis of fluoroquinolone resistance in clinical isolates of *Mycobacterium tuberculosis* from India [51].
Perria et al [52]	Perria et al reported on drug resistance pattern of Mycobacterium tuberculosis in seropositive and seronegative HIV-TB patients in Pune, India [52].
Trivedi and Desai [53]	Trivedi and Desai reported on primary antituberculosis drug resistance and acquired rifampicin resistance in Gujarat, India [53].
Hemvani et al [54]	Hemvani et al reported on drug resistance among tubercle bacilli from pulmonary tuberculosis cases in central India [54].

3. Mycobacterium Avium Complex Infection

Mycobacterium avium complex or atypical mycobacterial infection is a new emerging situation after the spreading of HIV [55 – 74]. This is primarily not a human infection but the poor immune status in HIV infected cases make affected human beings get this infection. This situation has been focused on in medicine and the problems can be seen around the world. This problem is also observed in India and, at present, is still a problem. Some important reports are presented in Table 4.

Table 4. Reports on *Mycobacterium avium* complex in India.

Author	Details
Venugopal et al [75]	Venugopal et al reported on drug resistance profile of human *Mycobacterium avium* complex strains from India [75].
Kamala et al [76]	Kamala et al reported on immune response and modulation of immune response induced in the guinea-pigs by reported on *Mycobacterium avium* complex and *Mycobacterium fortuitum* complex isolates from different sources in the south Indian BCG trial area [76].
Dam et al [77]	Dam et al reported on isolation of plasmids from *Mycobacterium avium* -intracellulare complex strains from India [77].
Kamala et al [78]	Kamala et al reported on isolation and Identification of Environmental Mycobacteria in the *Mycobacterium bovis* BCG Trial Area of South India [78].

References

[1] Grant A, Gothard P, Thwaites G. Managing drug resistant tuberculosis. *BMJ*. 2008 Aug 28;337:a1110.

[2] Jeong YJ, Lee KS. Pulmonary tuberculosis: up-to-date imaging and management. AJR *Am J Roentgenol*. 2008 Sep;191(3):834-44.

[3] Hernandez C, Cetner AS, Jordan JE, Puangsuvan SN, Robinson JK.Tuberculosis in the age of biologic therapy. *J Am Acad Dermatol*. 2008 Sep;59(3):363-80.

[4] McAdams HP, Erasmus J, Winter JA. Radiologic manifestations of pulmonary tuberculosis. *Radiol Clin North Am*. 1995 Jul;33(4):655-78.

[5] Okada M, Kobayashi K. Recent progress in mycobacteriology. *Kekkaku*. 2007 Oct;82(10):783-99.

[6] Yagi O, Kawabe Y, Nagayama N, Shimada M, Kawashima M, Kaneko Y, Ariga H, Ohshima N, Matsui Y, Suzuki J, Masuda K, Tamura A, Nagai H, Akagawa S, Machida K, Kurashima A, Nakajima Y, Yotsumoto H. Bone and joint tuberculosis concurrent with tuberculosis of other organs. *Kekkaku*. 2007 Jun;82(6):523-9.

[7] Yoshiyama T, Ogata H. CT screening before treatment of latent tuberculous infection for the diagnosis of clinical TB among contacts. *Kekkaku*. 2008 May;83(5):411-6.

[8] API Consensus Expert Committee. PI TB Consensus Guidelines 2006: Management of pulmonary tuberculosis, extra-pulmonary tuberculosis and tuberculosis in special situations. *J Assoc Physicians India*. 2006 Mar;54:219-34.

[9] Im JG, Itoh H, Shim YS, Lee JH, Ahn J, Han MC, Noma S. Pulmonary tuberculosis: CT findings--early active disease and sequential change with antituberculous therapy. *Radiology*. 1993 Mar;186(3):653-60.

[10] Abdel-Dayem HM, Naddaf S, Aziz M, Mina B, Turoglu T, Akisik MF, Omar WS, DiFabrizio L, LaBombardi V, Kempf JS. Sites of tuberculous involvement in patients with AIDS. Autopsy findings and evaluation of gallium imaging. *Clin Nucl Med*. 1997 May;22(5):310-4.

[11] Erokhin VV, Kornilova ZKh, Alekseeva LP. The specific features of the detection, clinical manifestations, and treatment of tuberculosis in the HIV-infected. *Probl Tuberk Bolezn Legk*. 2005;(10):20-8. Russian.

[12] Beigelman C, Sellami D, Brauner M. CT of parenchymal and bronchial tuberculosis. *Eur Radiol.* 2000;10(5):699-709.

[13] Hsieh SM, Hung CC, Chen MY, Chang SC, Hsueh PR, Luh KT, Chuang CY. Clinical features of tuberculosis associated with HIV infection in Taiwan. *J Formos Med Assoc.* 1996 Dec;95(12):923-8.

[14] Kim YI, Goo JM, Kim HY, Song JW, Im JG. Coexisting bronchogenic carcinoma and pulmonary tuberculosis in the same lobe: radiologic findings and clinical significance. *Korean J Radiol.* 2001 Jul-Sep;2(3):138-44.

[15] Tomioka H, Namba K. Development of antituberculous drugs: current status and future prospects. *Kekkaku*. 2006 Dec;81(12):753-74.

[16] Nyman RS, Brismar J, Hugosson C, Larsson SG, Lundstedt C. Imaging of tuberculosis--experience from 503 patients. I. Tuberculosis of the chest. *Acta Radiol.* 1996 Jul;37(4):482-8.

[17] Condos R, Rom WN, Schluger NW. Treatment of multidrug-resistant pulmonary tuberculosis with interferon-gamma via aerosol. *Lancet.* 1997 May 24;349(9064):1513-5.

[18] Leung AN, Brauner MW, Gamsu G, Mlika-Cabanne N, Ben Romdhane H, Carette MF, Grenier P. Pulmonary tuberculosis: comparison of CT findings in HIV-seropositive and HIV-seronegative patients. *Radiology.* 1996 Mar;198(3):687-91.

[19] Wang Q, Huang LL, Yue MG, Qin SL, Wang Y, Nie YX, Zhang CQ, Liang TJ, Zhao YM. 18F-FDG imaging by coincidence circuit SPECT with low-dose CT in preoperative assessment of pulmonary lesions. *Zhonghua Zhong Liu Za Zhi*. 2006 Dec;28(12):924-7.

[20] Poey C, Verhaegen F, Giron J, Lavayssiere J, Fajadet P, Duparc B. High resolution chest CT in tuberculosis: evolutive patterns and signs of activity. *J Comput Assist Tomogr.* 1997 Jul-Aug;21(4):601-7.

[21] Grant A, Gothard P, Thwaites G. Managing drug resistant tuberculosis. *BMJ.* 2008 Aug 28;337:a1110.

[22] Lalloo UG, Pillay S. Managing tuberculosis and HIV in sub-Sahara Africa.*Curr HIV/AIDS Rep*. 2008 Aug;5(3):132-9.

[23] Scarborough M, Thwaites GE. The diagnosis and management of acute bacterial meningitis in resource-poor settings. *Lancet Neurol.* 2008 Jul;7(7):637-48.

[24] Sousa M, Pozniak A, Boffito M. Pharmacokinetics and pharmacodynamics of drug interactions involving rifampicin, rifabutin and antimalarial drugs. *J Antimicrob Chemother.* 2008 Aug 18. [Epub ahead of print]

[25] Lew W, Pai M, Oxlade O, Martin D, Menzies D. Initial drug resistance and tuberculosis treatment outcomes: systematic review and meta-analysis. *Ann Intern Med.* 2008 Jul 15;149(2):123-34.

[26] Bhowruth V, Alderwick LJ, Brown AK, Bhatt A, Besra GS. Tuberculosis: a balanced diet of lipids and carbohydrates. *Biochem Soc Trans.* 2008 Aug;36(Pt 4):555-65.

[27] Méndez-Samperio P. Role of antimicrobial peptides in host defense against mycobacterial infections. *Peptides*. 2008 Oct;29(10):1836-41.

[28] Lew W, Pai M, Oxlade O, Martin D, Menzies D. Initial drug resistance and tuberculosis treatment outcomes: systematic review and meta-analysis. *Ann Intern Med.* 2008 Jul 15;149(2):123-34.

[29] Franke MF, Appleton SC, Bayona J, Arteaga F, Palacios E, Llaro K, Shin SS, Becerra MC, Murray MB, Mitnick CD. Risk factors and mortality associated with default from multidrug-resistant tuberculosis treatment. *Clin Infect Dis*. 2008 Jun 15;46(12):1844-51.

[30] Dover LG, Bhatt A, Bhowruth V, Willcox BE, Besra GS. New drugs and vaccines for drug-resistant Mycobacterium tuberculosis infections. *Expert Rev Vaccines*. 2008 May;7(4):481-97.

[31] Onyebujoh P, Zumla A, Ribeiro I, Rustomjee R, Mwaba P, Gomes M, Grange JM. Treatment of tuberculosis: present status and future prospects. *Bull World Health Organ*. 2005;83:857-65.

[32] Silva CL, Faccioli LH, Rocha GM. The role of cachectin/TNF in the pathogenesis of tuberculosis. *Braz J Med Biol Res*. 1988;21:489-92.

[33] Zhang M, Wang JD, Li ZF, Xie J, Yang YP, Zhong Y, Wang HH. Expression and characterization of the carboxyl esterase Rv3487c from Mycobacterium tuberculosis. *Protein Expr Purif*. 2005;42:59-66.

[34] Kovalev GK. Differentiation of Mycobacteria. *Klin Lab Diagn*. 1993;(3):71-3.

[35] Khan S, Situ G, Decker K, Schmidt CJ. GoFigure: automated Gene Ontology annotation. *Bioinformatics* 2003;19:2484-5.

[36] Talati S, Mahadevan PR. Lipase activity in Mycobacterium leprae--an indicator of metabolic function. *Indian J Lepr*. 1986;58:367-72.

[37] Saviola B, Woolwine SC, Bishai WR. Isolation of acid-inducible genes of Mycobacterium tuberculosis with the use of recombinase-based in vivo expression technology. *Infect Immun*. 2003;71:1379-88.

[38] Williams BG, Granich R, Chauhan LS, Dharmshaktu NS, Dye C. The impact of HIV/AIDS on the control of tuberculosis in India. *Proc Natl Acad Sci U S A*. 2005 Jul 5;102(27):9619-24.

[39] Murali MS, Sajjan BS. DOTS strategy for control of tuberculosis epidemic. *Indian J Med Sci*. 2002 Jan;56(1):16-8.

[40] Karande S, Bavdekar SB. Children and multidrug-resistant tuberculosis in Mumbai (Bombay), India. *Emerg Infect Dis*. 2002 Nov;8(11):1360-1

[41] Balasubramanian VN, Oommen K, Samuel R. DOT or not? Direct observation of anti-tuberculosis treatment and patient outcomes, Kerala State, India. *Int J Tuberc Lung Dis*. 2000 May;4(5):409-13.

[42] Sawert H. The re-emergence of tuberculosis and its economic implications. *Pharmacoeconomics*. 1996 May;9(5):379-81.

[43] Mondal R, Jain A. Extensively drug-resistant Mycobacterium tuberculosis, India. *Emerg Infect Dis*. 2007 Sep;13(9):1429-31.

[44] Almeida D, Rodrigues C, Ashavaid TF, Lalvani A, Udwadia ZF, Mehta A. High incidence of the Beijing genotype among multidrug-resistant isolates of Mycobacterium tuberculosis in a tertiary care center in Mumbai, India. *Clin Infect Dis*. 2005 Mar 15;40(6):881-6.

[45] Suresh N, Singh UB, Arora J, Pant H, Seth P, Sola C, Rastogi N, Samantaray JC, Pande JN. rpoB gene sequencing and spoligotyping of multidrug-resistant Mycobacterium tuberculosis isolates from India. *Infect Genet Evol*. 2006 Nov;6(6):474-83.

[46] Singh S, Sankar MM, Gopinath K. High rate of extensively drug-resistant tuberculosis in Indian AIDS patients. *AIDS*. 2007 Nov 12;21(17):2345-7.

[47] Mistry NF, Iyer AM, D'souza DT, Taylor GM, Young DB, Antia NH. Spoligotyping of Mycobacterium tuberculosis isolates from multiple-drug-resistant tuberculosis patients from Bombay, India. *J Clin Microbiol.* 2002 Jul;40(7):2677-80.

[48] Almeida D, Rodrigues C, Udwadia ZF, Lalvani A, Gothi GD, Mehta P, Mehta A. Incidence of multidrug-resistant tuberculosis in urban and rural India and implications for prevention. *Clin Infect Dis.* 2003 Jun 15;36(12):e152-4.

[49] Harris KA Jr, Mukundan U, Musser JM, Kreiswirth BN, Lalitha MK. Genetic diversity and evidence for acquired antimicrobial resistance in Mycobacterium tuberculosis at a large hospital in South India. *Int J Infect Dis.* 2000;4(3):140-7.

[50] Mahajan M, Agarwal DS, Gadre DJ, Singh NP, Gupta HC, Talwar V. Initial and acquired drug resistance of Mycobacterium tuberculosis in east Delhi. *J Commun Dis.* 1996 Mar;28(1):15-9.

[51] Sulochana S, Narayanan S, Paramasivan CN, Suganthi C, Narayanan PR. Analysis of fluoroquinolone resistance in clinical isolates of Mycobacterium tuberculosis from India. *J Chemother.* 2007 Apr;19(2):166-71.

[52] Perria M, Tripathy S, Inamdar V, Ramesh K, Bhavsar M, Date A, Iyyer R, Acchammachary A, Mehendale S, Risbud A. Drug resistance pattern of Mycobacterium tuberculosis in seropositive and seronegative HIV-TB patients in Pune, India. Indian *J Med Res.* 2005 Apr;121(4):235-9.

[53] Trivedi SS, Desai SG. Primary antituberculosis drug resistance and acquired rifampicin resistance in Gujarat, India. *Tubercle.* 1988 Mar;69(1):37-42.

[54] Hemvani N, Chitnis DS, Bhatia GC, Sharma N. Drug resistance among tubercle bacilli from pulmonary tuberculosis cases in central India. *Indian J Med Sci.* 2001 Jul;55(7):382-92.

[55] Corti M, Palmero D. Mycobacterium avium complex infection in HIV/AIDS patients. *Expert Rev Anti Infect Ther.* 2008 Jun;6(3):351-63.

[56] Lange CG, Woolley IJ, Brodt RH. Disseminated mycobacterium avium-intracellulare complex (MAC) infection in the era of effective antiretroviral therapy: is prophylaxis still indicated? *Drugs.* 2004;64(7):679-92.

[57] Karakousis PC, Moore RD, Chaisson RE. Mycobacterium avium complex in patients with HIV infection in the era of highly active antiretroviral therapy. *Lancet Infect Dis.* 2004 Sep;4(9):557-65.

[58] Phillips P, Chan K, Hogg R, Bessuille E, Black W, Talbot J, O'Shaughnessy M, Montaner J. Azithromycin prophylaxis for Mycobacterium avium complex during the era of highly active antiretroviral therapy: evaluation of a provincial program. *Clin Infect Dis.* 2002 Feb 1;34(3):371-8. Epub 2001 Dec 14.

[59] Tumbarello M, Tacconelli E, de Donati KG, Bertagnolio S, Longo B, Ardito F, Fadda G, Cauda R. Changes in incidence and risk factors of Mycobacterium avium complex infections in patients with AIDS in the era of new antiretroviral therapies. *Eur J Clin Microbiol Infect Dis.* 2001 Jul;20(7):498-501.

[60] Baril L, Jouan M, Agher R, Cambau E, Caumes E, Bricaire F, Katlama C. Impact of highly active antiretroviral therapy on onset of Mycobacterium avium complex infection and cytomegalovirus disease in patients with AIDS. *AIDS.* 2000 Nov 10;14(16):2593-6.

[61] Aberg JA, Williams PL, Liu T, Lederman HM, Hafner R, Torriani FJ, Lennox JL, Dube MP, MacGregor RR, Currier JS; AIDS Clinical Trial Group 393 Study Team. A study of discontinuing maintenance therapy in human immunodeficiency virus-infected

subjects with disseminated Mycobacterium avium complex: AIDS Clinical Trial Group 393 Study Team. *J Infect Dis*. 2003 Apr 1;187(7):1046-52.

[62] Lazaro E, Coureau G, Guedj J, Blanco P, Pellegrin I, Commenges D, Dabis F, Moreau JF, Pellegrin JL, Thiébaut R; ANRS Co3 Aquitaine Cohort. Change in T-lymphocyte count after initiation of highly active antiretroviral therapy in HIV-infected patients with history of Mycobacterium avium complex infection. *Antivir Ther*. 2006;11(3):343-50.

[63] Zeller V, Truffot C, Agher R, Bossi P, Tubiana R, Caumes E, Jouan M, Bricaire F, Katlama C. Discontinuation of secondary prophylaxis against disseminated Mycobacterium avium complex infection and toxoplasmic encephalitis. *Clin Infect Dis*. 2002 Mar 1;34(5):662-7.

[64] Aberg JA, Chin-Hong PV, McCutchan A, Koletar SL, Currier JS. Localized osteomyelitis due to Mycobacterium avium complex in patients with Human Immunodeficiency Virus receiving highly active antiretroviral therapy. *Clin Infect Dis*. 2002 Jul 1;35(1):E8-E13.

[65] Havlir DV, Torriani FJ, Schrier RD, Huang JY, Lederman MM, Chervenak KA, Boom WH. Serum interleukin-6 (IL-6), IL-10, tumor necrosis factor (TNF) alpha, soluble type II TNF receptor, and transforming growth factor beta levels in human immunodeficiency virus type 1-infected individuals with Mycobacterium avium complex disease. *J Clin Microbiol*. 2001 Jan;39(1):298-303.

[66] Girmenia C, Martino P, Mazzucconi MG, Bizzoni L, Cassone A. HAART and Mycobacterium avium complex in an HIV infected patient with severe factor VII deficiency. *Haemophilia*. 2000 Mar;6(2):116-7.

[67] Sesin GP, Manzi SF, Pacheco R. New trends in the drug therapy of localized and disseminated Mycobacterium avium complex infection. *Am J Health Syst Pharm*. 1996 Nov 1;53(21):2585-90.

[68] Shafran SD, Mashinter LD, Phillips P, Lalonde RG, Gill MJ, Walmsley SL, Toma E, Conway B, Fong IW, Rachlis AR, Williams KE, Garber GE, Schlech WF, Smaill F, Pradier C. Successful discontinuation of therapy for disseminated Mycobacterium avium complex infection after effective antiretroviral therapy. *Ann Intern Med*. 2002 Nov 5;137(9):734-7.

[69] Sterling TR, Moore RD, Graham NM, Astemborski J, Vlahov D, Chaisson RE.Mycobacterium tuberculosis infection and disease are not associated with protection against subsequent disseminated M. avium complex disease. *AIDS*.1998 Aug 20;12(12):1451-7.

[70] Dautzenberg B. Rationale for the prevention of disseminated Mycobacterium avium-intracellulare complex disease. *Drugs*. 1997;54 Suppl 2:1-7.

[71] Desimone JA Jr, Babinchak TJ, Kaulback KR, Pomerantz RJ. Treatment of Mycobacterium avium complex immune reconstitution disease in HIV-1-infected individuals. *AIDS Patient Care STDS*. 2003 Dec;17(12):617-22.

[72] Sendi PP, Craig BA, Meier G, Pfluger D, Gafni A, Opravil M, Battegay M, Bucher HC. Cost-effectiveness of azithromycin for preventing Mycobacterium avium complex infection in HIV-positive patients in the era of highly active antiretroviral therapy.The Swiss HIV Cohort Study. *J Antimicrob Chemother*. 1999 Dec;44(6):811-7.

[73] Rossi M, Flepp M, Telenti A, Schiffer V, Egloff N, Bucher H, Vernazza P, Bernasconi E, Weber R, Rickenbach M, Furrer H; Swiss HIV Cohort Study Disseminated M. avium complex infection in the Swiss HIV Cohort Study: declining incidence,

improved prognosis and discontinuation of maintenance therapy. *Swiss Med Wkly.* 2001 Aug 11;131(31-32):471-7.

[74] Prevention strategies for Mycobacterium avium-intracellulare complex (MAC) infection. A review of recent studies in patients with AIDS. *Drugs.* 1997;54 Suppl 2:8-15.

[75] Venugopal D, Kumar S, Isa M, Bose M. Drug resistance profile of human Mycobacterium avium complex strains from India. *Indian J Med Microbiol.* 2007 Apr;25(2):115-20.

[76] Kamala T, Paramasivan CN, Herbert D, Venkatesan P, Prabhakar R. Immune response & modulation of immune response induced in the guinea-pigs by Mycobacterium avium complex (MAC) & M. fortuitum complex isolates from different sources in the south Indian BCG trial area. *Indian J Med Res.* 1996 Apr;103:201-11.

[77] Dam T, Bose M, Isa M, Virdi JS. Isolation of plasmids from Mycobacterium avium-intracellulare complex (MAC) strains from India.*J Med Microbiol.* 2000 Apr;49(4):392-4.

[78] Kamala T, Paramasivan CN, Herbert D, Venkatesan P, Prabhakar R. Isolation and Identification of Environmental Mycobacteria in the Mycobacterium bovis BCG Trial Area of South India. *Appl Environ Microbiol.* 1994 Jun;60(6):2180-2183.

Chapter XI

A Study of Anal and Perianal Tubercular Infection

PJ Gupta*

Gupta Nursing Home, D/9, Laxminagar, NAGPUR- 440022 India

Abstract

Anal tuberculosis is not an uncommon pathology found in the tropics. A tuberculous origin must be considered when the cause of perianal lesion is unclear to avoid undesirable delay in the diagnosis and treatment of this disease. This brief treatise explores the different etiopathogenic, clinical, and diagnostic manifestations of ano-perianal tuberculosis.

Introduction

Tuberculosis around the anus is a rare extra pulmonary form of the disease [1]. There is a need to recognize its presence because it calls for a specific treatment. Tuberculosis can affect any part of the gastrointestinal tract, (GIT) from the esophagus to the anal canal. Though tuberculosis of the GIT is frequently encountered in tropical countries, tuberculosis of bowel distal to ileocaecal junction is rare and is rarely considered as a differential diagnosis of proctological disorders [2].

Tuberculosis of the gastrointestinal tract may be primary or secondary to a primary focus elsewhere [3]. Primary intestinal tuberculosis is attributed to bovine tubercle bacilli entering the system through milk intake. The incidence of primary tuberculosis is on the decline due to public preference for pasteurized milk.

* Consulting Proctologist, Gupta Nursing Home, D/9, Laxminagar, NAGPUR- 440022 India

While the rate of patients with extra pulmonary tuberculosis has increased in the last few years (about 5% of all cases) with display of a wide spectrum of its clinical manifestations, the anal localization still is a rare occurrence (0.7%) according to available published data [4].

The most frequently encountered anorectal tuberculous lesions are suppurations and fistulae [5]. Tuberculosis is a neglected cause of anal sepsis, not often recognized, and therefore does not get the desired treatment.

The presentation of the disease may take many forms, with an atypical and uncharacteristic clinical picture, which makes it difficult to diagnose them preoperatively. A few of the presenting features of ano-perianal tuberculosis could be summarized here-

Table 1.- Symptomatology of ano-perianal tuberculosis.

1. Anal pain, fever and cough [6].
2. Anal or perianal ulcer with purulent exudates.
3. A non-healing wound around the anus [7].
4. Anal fistula [8] [Usually recurrent with multiple external openings, gross scarring and induration]
5. Perianal cutaneous ulcerations [9].
6. Acute perianal abscess [10].
7. Bleeding anal ulcer [11].
8. Anal stricture [12].
9. Hemorrhoidal thrombosis with fever and purulent discharge [13].
10. As an associated anal lesion with HIV positive patient [14].

A good digital examination is usually sufficient to diagnosis anal fistulae. Nearly all fistulas are complex and secondary tracks or additional complicating features are common, even at first presentation [15]. Clinically, patients with anal tuberculosis may present as growth and simulate carcinoma. These patients may present with bleeding per-rectum and pain while passing stools. Anal fissures occur in an unusual location, which is slow to heal, and should be appropriately screened to rule out tuberculous disease.

Tuberculosis can be a part of the complicating infection of HIV-positive patients. Anal tubercular sepsis seems to have characteristic clinical features. It should be considered in cases of known pulmonary or extra pulmonary tuberculosis or if anal sepsis is persistent, recurrent, or complex in nature [15].

Various Forms of Ano-Perianal Tuberculosis

Tuberculosis is known to manifest through many atypical and unexpected clinical presentations. These variables are also seen in the proctology practice. Few of the unusual forms of the lesion reported are as follows-

Table 2. - Varied presentations of ano-perianal tuberculosis.

- **Pilonidal sinus [16] (Figure 1)**
- **Fistula in ano (Figure 2)**
- **Anal ulceration with inguinal adenopathy [17]**
- **Non healing ulcer at the anal orifice [18]**
- **Recurrent perianal growth (Tuberculosis verrucosa cutis) [19]**
- **Rectal stricture [20]**
- **Anal fistula with tubercular epididymitis [21]**
- **Anal fistula with tubercular salpingitis [22]**
- **Anal fissure [23] (Figure 3)**
- **Associated with malignancy of anal canal [24]**
- **Varicose anorectal tuberculosis [25]**
- **Atypically localized scrofuloderma [26]**
- **Anal stricture [27]**
- **Rectal submucosal tumor [28]**

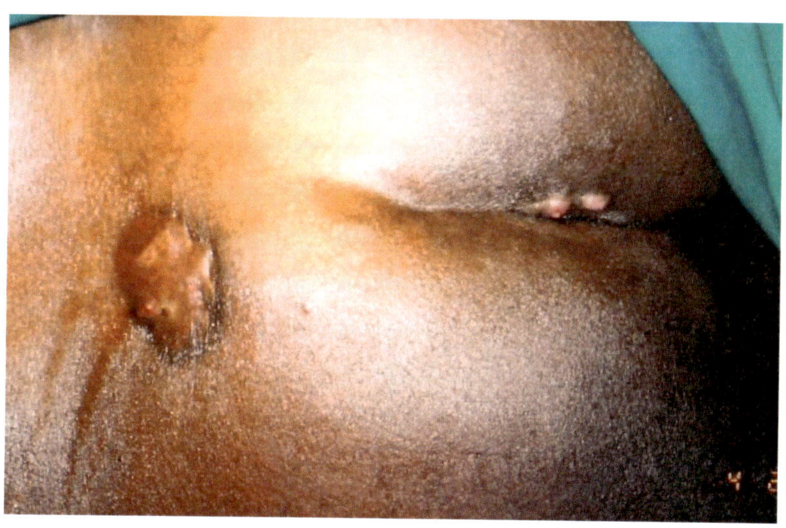

Figure 1- Tubercular pilonidal sinus.

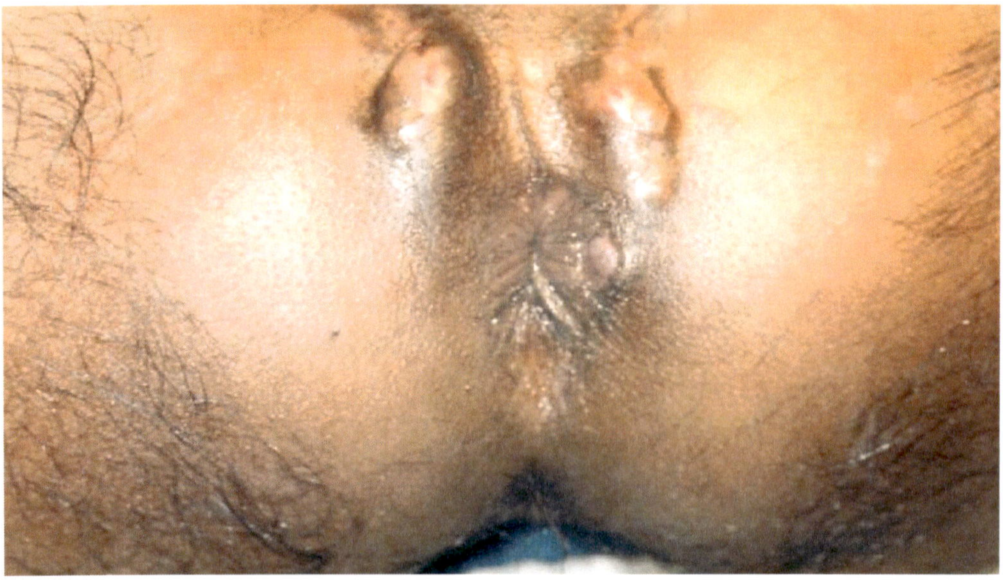

Figure 2. Tubercular fistulae in ano.

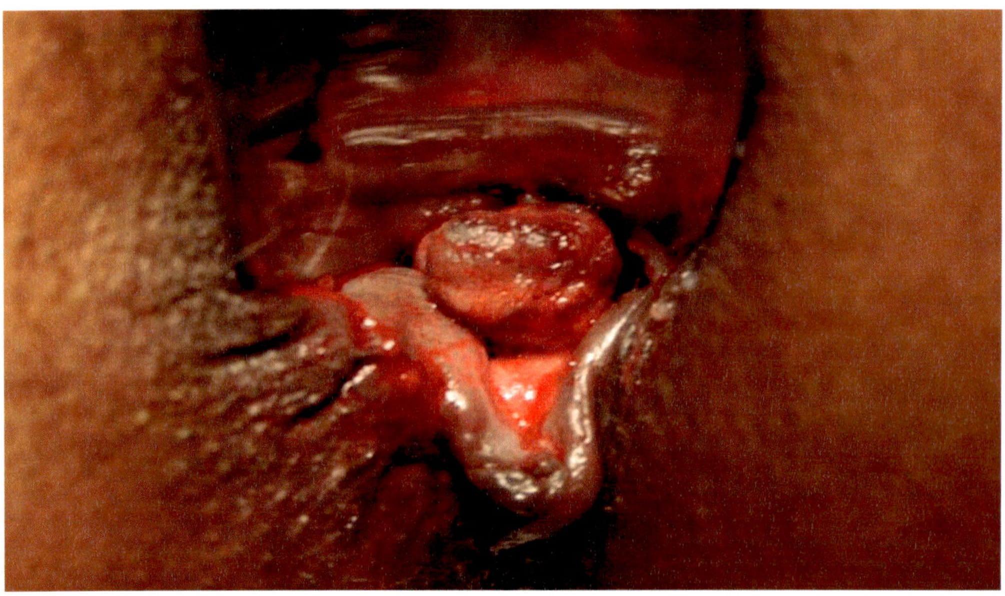

Figure 3. Tubercular granuloma of the anal canal with anal fissure.

Investigations

Despite the availability of several tests, early diagnosis of anal and perianal tuberculosis remains a challenge. In countries like India, the search begins with the routine tests as total leucocytes count, Erythrocyte Sedimentation Rate, Mantoux test, detection of acid-fast bacilli in the discharge or tissue section from the lesion. Thorough investigation could be needed to establish the presence of pulmonary tuberculosis. Clinical diagnosis is usually dependent on microscopic detection using Ziehl-Neelsen stain [6] and mycobacterial culture [7], but the sensitivity and specificity of these two methods are low. So, tests that are more specific are needed to come to a definite conclusion. A battery of investigative tools listed below is available to accurately diagnose the disease.

Table 3. Investigation protocol for detection of ano-perianal tuberculosis.

1. **Culture**
2. **Biopsy [29]**
3. **Examination of discharge for Acid Fast Bacilli**
4. **Fine needle aspiration cytology [30]**
5. **Mantoux test**
6. **ELISA test [31-32] (Tuberculosis IgA EIA, Pathozyme-TB complex, Pathozyme – Myco IgG, Pathozyme -Myco IgA, and Pathozyme -Myco IgM) to detect antibodies against Mycobacteria**
7. **Computerized Tomography [28]**
8. **Magnetic Resonance Imaging [33]**
9. **Fistulogram [8]**
10. **Molicular diagnosis by nested polymerase chain reaction [34]**
11. **Percutaneous transperineal sonography [35]**
12. **Rapid Immunochromatographic assay [36] (ICT Tuberculosis)**

The serodiagnosis of tuberculosis has long been the subject of controversy, as we still lack a test with widespread clinical utility. The poor sensitivity and specificity of commercial assays preclude their use as the sole means of diagnosis. All these assays use mycobacterial antigens adsorbed onto a surface. There is a high possibility of false positive and false negative reactions [31]. The overall sensitivity of these tests for extra pulmonary tuberculosis is as low as 16.7% [32].

The relatively low sensitivities and specificities of these serologic tests make them poor tools for the diagnosis of tuberculosis. For the EIA-IgA, the sensitivity reported was 74% and the specificity was 68% when a cutoff determined by a receiver operator characteristic curve was used. For the EIA-IgG, the sensitivity was 69% and the specificity was 64% [37].

The simplest rapid method for diagnosis of the disease, perhaps, is the detection of acid-fast bacilli by microscopy. However, 75% of patients with extra pulmonary tubercular disease are smear negative, and in the situation even contemporary culture methods might take several weeks to become positive [34].

Histological examination of the excised fistula is mandatory for the diagnosis of anal tuberculosis. In other perianal pathologies, ridge biopsies of the growth or histopathological study of excised lesion helps in clinching the diagnosis [5, 7,16].

Experience shows that a triad of FNAC, AFB smear, and culture are cheaper, foolproof, and confirmatory when compared to costlier tests like TB IgG, IgM, or ICT tests [30].

Differential Diagnosis

Perianal cutaneous ulcerations in tropical countries have multiple causes: bacterial, viral, and parasitic. Infections, such as amoebiasis and actinomycosis have to be explored in priority [9]. Emphasis should be put on the diversity of clinical presentations including acute perianal abscess, chronic anal ulcer, and fistula in ano. Because of nonspecific symptoms and non-characteristic radiological and endoscopic features, the diagnosis of tuberculosis rests mainly on histological evidence of the classical tubercle in a surgical biopsy specimen. Crohn's disease and tuberculosis pose major diagnostic problems for clinicians where these conditions coexist [38]. The necessity of careful study in differentiating the lesions from carcinoma could not be overemphasized. Few other clinical conditions mimicking tuberculosis are-

Table 4. Differential diagnosis of ano-perianal tuberculosis.

- **Hidradinitis suppurative [39]**
- **Bartholinitis**
- **Radiation injuries**
- **Lymphoma**
- **Antibiomas**

Discussion

Though tuberculous involvement of the anus is declining as the result of BCG-vaccination, awareness about personal hygiene and improvement of public health; it still is one of the commonest causes of granulomatous diseases within the anorectal region [1].

It is speculated that the tuberculous anal lesions in few patients are caused by the dissemination from the pulmonary focus via the hematogeneous and lymphogeneous routes, while in few others; the lesion may be present in the gastrointestinal tract and rectum [6]. A high index of suspicion is important to ensure an early diagnosis. Treatment of tubercular lesions of the anus should include conventional surgical treatment of anal sepsis and specific medical anti-tuberculosis treatment [40]. Antitubercular drugs have changed the dismal outlook for patients with ano-perianal tuberculosis. They also have been made surgery safe and often curative. In most of the situations, the patients are treated with four drug antitubercular chemotherapy [4]. It can be concluded that a tuberculous origin must be considered when the cause of anal and perianal lesions is unclear or when it presents recurrently. Similarly, patients having perianal sepsis and a concurrent tubercular lesion elsewhere should be suspected to have a tubercular origin to avoid undesirable delays in the diagnosis and treatment of this disease [2].

References

[1] Romelaer C, Abramowitz L. Anal abscess with a tuberculous origin: report of two cases and review of the literature. *Gastroenterol Clin Biol.* 2007; 31(1): 94-6.

[2] Chung CC, Choi CL, Kwok SP, Leung KL, Lau WY, Li AK. Anal and perianal tuberculosis: a report of three cases in 10 years. *J R Coll Surg Edinb.* 1997; 42:189-190.Iwase A, Shiota S, Nakaya Y, Sakamoto K, Aoki S, Matsuoka R, Nagayama T. An autopsy case of severe tuberculosis associated with anal fistula and intestinal perforation. *Kekkaku.* 1997; 72: 515-518.

[3] Tan KK, Chen K, Sim R.The Spectrum of Abdominal Tuberculosis in a Developed Country: A Single Institution's Experience Over 7 Years.*J Gastrointest Surg.* 2008 Sep 3.

[4] Fernández Rivero JM, Rocha Ramírez JL, Villanueva Sáenz E, Sierra Montenegro E, Rojas Illanes M. Anorectal tuberculosis. Case report. *Rev Gastroenterol Mex.* 2007; 72(1): 40-2.

[5] Gierthmühlen M, Laiffer G, Viehl CT, Savic S, Bremerich J, Mueller C, Christ M. No ordinary anal fistula. *Internist* (Berl). 2008; 49(4): 490, 492-4.

[6] Ohse H, Ishii Y, Saito T, Watanabe S, Fukai S, Yanai N, Tamai N, Monma Y, Hasegawa S.A case of pulmonary tuberculosis associated with tuberculous fistula of anus] *Kekkaku.*1995; 70: 385-388.

[7] Gupta PJ. A case of multiple (eight external openings) tubercular anal fistulae. Case report. *Eur Rev Med Pharmacol Sci.* 2007; 11(5): 359-61.

[8] Bokhari I, Shah SS, Inamullah, Mehmood Z, Ali SU, Khan A. Tubercular fistula-in-ano. *J Coll Physicians Surg Pak.* 2008; 18(7): 401-3.

[9] O'Donohoe MK, Waldron RP, O'Malley E. Miliary tuberculosis presenting as an acute perianal abscess. Report of a case. *Dis Colon Rectum.* 1987; 30:697-698.

[10] Candela F, Serrano P, Arriero JM, Teruel A, Reyes D, Calpena R. Perianal disease of tuberculous origin: report of a case and review of the literature. *Dis Colon Rectum.*1999; 42:110-112.

[11] Hajji A, Abbar M, el Kirat-Hajji Z, Derouiche A, Moulay A. Anal and perianal tuberculosis. Apropos of 15 cases. *Chirurgie.* 1987; 113:793-802.

[12] Borki K, Saissy JM, Benomar S, Okheira H, Dimou M, Ducourau JP. Anorectal tuberculosis disclosed by hemorrhoidal thrombosis. *Med Trop* (Mars). 1986; 46:75-77.

[13] Musch E, Tunnerhoff-Mucke A. Tuberculous anal fistula in acquired immunologic deficiency syndrome. *Z Gastroenterol*. 1995; 33:440-444.

[14] Kraemer M, Gill SS, Seow-Choen F. Tuberculous anal sepsis: report of clinical features in 20 cases. *Dis Colon Rectum*. 2000; 43:1589-1591.

[15] Wang JP, Ding WX, Deng YH, Lan P, Pan K, Dong GH, Deng JZ, Wang L, Wu XJ, Guo XF, Zheng J. Preoperative chemoradiotherapy with FOLFOX in low rectal cancer: a multicenter study. *Zhonghua Wei Chang Wai Ke Za Zhi*. 2008; 11(2): 116-9.

[16] Nalepa P, Pasowicz M, Straczek C. Tuberculosis ulcerosa of the anus and anal fissure accompanied by pulmonary tuberculosis. *Pol Merkur Lekarski*. 2006; 21(125): 477-9.

[17] Gonzalez Moran A, Chaves Sanchez F, Aramendi Sanchez T, Carbonero Diaz P, Colomer Rosas A. Tuberculosis of the perianal orifice. *Rev Clin Esp*. 1988; 183:52-53.

[18] Sayal SK, Falleiro JJ, Motwani H, Rao VS. Tuberculosis verrucosa cutis (a case report). *Indian J Dermatol*. 1989; 34:17-20.

[19] Das PC, Radhakrishna K, Rao PL. Rectal stricture: a complication of tuberculosis. *J Pediatr Surg*. 1996; 31:983-984.

[20] Williams JG, Farrands PA, Williams AB, Taylor BA, Lunniss PJ, Sagar PM, Varma JS, George BD.The treatment of anal fistula: ACPGBI position statement. *Colorectal Dis*. 2007; 9 Suppl 4:18-50.

[21] Akgun E, Tekin F, Ersin S, Osmanoglu H.Isolated perianal tuberculosis. *Neth J Med*. 2005; 63(3): 115-7.

[22] Myers SR. Tuberculous fissure-in ano. *J R Soc Med*. 1994; 87:46

[23] Sarela AI, Supe AN. Tuberculous perianal ulcers. *J R Soc Med*. 1996; 89:584.

[24] Fulton JO, Lazarus C. Varicose anorectal tuberculosis. A case report. *S Afr Med J*. 1987; 71:108-109.

[25] Polakova K. Atypically localized scrofuloderma. *Bratisl Lek Listy*. 1993; 94:536-538.

[26] Kato K, Shudo H, Makihara S. Anal stricture caused by tuberculosis. *Shujutsu*. 1967; 21:107-110.

[27] Yanagida T, Oya M, Iwase N, Okuyama T, Terada H, Sasaki K, Akao S, Ishikawa H, Satoh H. Rectal submucosal tumor-like lesion originating from intestinal tuberculosis. *J Gastroenterol*. 1997; 32:822-825.

[28] Shukla HS, Gupta SC, Singh G, Singh PA. Tubercular fistula in ano. Br *J Surg*.1988; 75:38-39.

[29] Sinha SK, Chatterjee M, Bhattacharya S, Pathak SK, Mitra RB, Karak K, Mukherjee M. Diagnostic evaluation of extrapulmonary tuberculosis by fine needle aspiraton (FNA) supplemented with AFB smear and culture. *J Indian Med Assoc*. 2003; 101: 590-591.

[30] Pereira Arias-Bouda LM, Kuijper S, van Deutekom H, van Gijlswijk R, Pekel I, Jansen HM, Kolk AH. Enzyme-linked immunosorbent assays using immune complexes for the diagnosis of tuberculosis. *J Immunol Methods* 2003; 283: 115-124.

[31] Sudha Pottumarthy S, Virginia C. Wells VC, Morris AJ. A Comparison of Seven Tests for Serological Diagnosis of Tuberculosis. *J Clin Microbiol* 2000; 38:2227-2231.

[32] Cuenod CA, de Parades V, Siauve N, Marteau P, Grataloup C, Hernigou A, Berger A, Cugnenc PH, Frija G. MR imaging of ano-perineal suppurations. *J Radiol* 2003; 84:516-528.

[33] Shan YS, Yan JJ, Sy ED, Jin YT, Lee JC. Nested polymerase chain reaction in the diagnosis of negative Ziehl-Neelsen stained Mycobacterium tuberculosis fistula-in-ano: report of four cases. *Dis Colon Rectum*. 2002; 45:1685-1688.

[34] Bonatti H, Lugger P, Hechenleitner P, Oberwalder M, Kafka-Ritsch R, Conrad F, Aigner F, Mallouhi A, Bodner G. Transperineal sonography in anorectal disorders. *Ultraschall Med.* 2004; 25:111-115.

[35] Bartoloni A, Strohmeyer M, Bartalesi F, Messeri D, Tortoli E, Farese A, Leoncini F, Nutini S, Righi R, Gabbuti A, Mazzotta F, Paradisi F. Evaluation of a rapid immunochromatographic test for the serologic diagnosis of tuberculosis in Italy. *Clin Microbiol Infect*. 2003; 9: 632-639.

[36] Conde MB, Suffys P, Lapa E, Silva JR, Kritski AL, Dorman.SE. Immunoglobulin A (IgA) and IgG Immune Responses against P-90 Antigen for Diagnosis of Pulmonary Tuberculosis and Screening for Mycobacterium tuberculosis Infection. *Clin Diagn Immunol* 2004; 11: 94-97.

[37] Jayanthi V, Robinson RJ, Malathi S, Rani B, Balambal R, Chari S, Taghuram K, Madanagopalan N, Mayberry JF. Does Crohn's disease need differentiation from tuberculosis? *J Gastroenterol Hepatol.* 1996; 11:183-186.Sharma MP, Bhatia V.Abdominal tuberculosis. *Indian J Med Res*. 2004 Oct; 120(4): 305-15.

[38] Alyoune M, Nadir S, Merzouk M, Mounadif A, Biadillah MC, Jamil D, Alaoui R, Cherkaoui A. Tuberculous anal fistulas. 13 cases. *Ann Gastroenterol Hepatol (Paris)* 1994; 30:9-11.

Chapter XII

Cutaneous Tuberculosis – A Review

L.Padmavathy[1] and L. Lakshmana Rao[2]
[1]Urban Health Center, Division of Community Medicine
[2] Division of Pathology, Rajah Muthiah Medical College,
Annamalai University, Annamalai Nagar, Tamil Nadu, India

Introduction

From time immemorial, the two mycobacterial diseases tuberculosis and leprosy have ranked amongst the most feared and dreaded diseases that afflict mankind. The genus Mycobacterium is responsible for more misery and suffering than any other genus of bacteria. Tuberculosis was dubbed by the evangelist John Bunyan as "the captain of all these men of death". It was also known as "Rajayakshma", which means 'the king of diseases', while leprosy, caused by *Mycobacterium leprae* is termed the 'disease of kings' [1]

Also known as the "white plague", tuberculosis kills and cripples millions of people. This disease represents a dynamic balance between man and *Mycobacterium tuberculosis.* [2] It is now the foremost cause of death from a single infectious agent in the world [3]

The earliest tangible record of pulmonary tuberculosis is the clay tablet inscription from the library of the Assyrian king Assurbanipal (668 to 626 BC) [4].

The Hindus called this disease, *sosha* (cough) or *rajayakshma* (wasting). The Greeks named it *phthisis* (to waste), and in Roman times this condition was *tabes* (a near equivalent to *phthisis*). Once the English speaking world developed, the familiar term consumption – derived from the Latin *consumere* (to consume or wear away) - entered the literature.

Greek literature contains numerous references to conditions resembling consumption, for example by Homer (800 BC). Hippocrates (460-377 BC) probably introduced the term *phthisis* and described the appearance of consumption as languorous, emaciated and physically debilitated, with red cheeks. Aristotle (382-322 BC) recognized the contagious nature of the disorder. Plato (430-347 BC) recommended no treatment because caring for the chronic tuberculosis patients was of no advantage to the patient or to the state. Galen (131-

200 AD) practising in Rome, noticed the contagious nature of phthisis. During the dark ages (400-1400B.C.), all knowledge of the disease was lost. Touching the King's feet for the cure of 'King's Evil' (as tuberculosis disease was then known), was prevalent during the eleventh and twelfth centuries in England and elsewhere. In Britain, Edward the confessor (1004-1066 AD) exercised the right of touching the tuberculosis patients for the relief of the 'King's evil'. Queen Anne was the last English ruler who practiced quack medicine for the treatment of 'King's evil' [4]

The turning point in the history of tuberculosis occurred at a meeting of the Berlin Physiological society on the evening of 24th March 1882, when Robert Koch, described the isolation of the causative organism of that disease. In 1868, Jean-Antoine Villemin, a French military surgeon, established the communicable nature of this disease by experimental transmission to rabbits. Theobald Smith (1898) isolated the bovine bacillus. In December 1890, Koch produced tuberculin and described 'Koch's Phenomenon. [5] In 1896, Lehman and Newmann assigned the term 'mycobacterium', to the genus, to describe the mould-like pellicle formed by M.tuberculosis when grown on liquid media.

A vaccine was produced by Calmette and Guerin, after passaging a supposedly bovine tubercle bacillus 230 times on potato slices soaked in bile and glycerol over a period of 13 years. In July 1921, this vaccine Bacille Calmette–Guerin (BCG) was first administered to a newborn whose grand mother had tuberculosis. It is the only vaccine against tuberculosis, currently in use worldwide.

Development of an acid-fast stain by Ehrlich (1885) and the discovery of X-Rays by Roentgen, in 1895 facilitated a more accurate diagnosis of tuberculosis.

A new era of chemotherapy dawned in 1944 when Schwartz Bugie and Waksman reported their discovery of streptomycin and its efficacy against *Mycobacterium tuberculosis* and other related species. Since the introduction of streptomycin, several synthetic antimicrobials and antibiotics have been discovered from time to time. The use of rifampicin in association with Isoniazid (INAH) as a primary therapy has revolutionized and shortened the duration of the treatment.

With the introduction of many public health measures and chemotherapy during the second half of this century, there was a dramatic decline in the morbidity and mortality, due to tuberculosis. .

However, tuberculosis actually is on the rise again,[6] especially among the homeless, alcohol and drug abuse population and the AIDS patients. The increasing number of multi-drug resistant strains of *Mycobacterium tuberculosis* isolates from both AIDS and non-AIDS patients is an ominous trend that threatens tuberculosis eradication programmes worldwide.

Cutaneous Tuberculosis

Tuberculosis can affect any organ or tissue in the body and the dermatological manifestations constitute a minor proportion. Cutaneous tuberculosis, especially lupus vulgaris were described repeatedly in the seventeenth and eighteenth centuries and the word "lupus "was used by some of the early authors. Bayle was the first to discover that tuberculosis was not confined to the lungs but could affect the whole body. Erasmus Wilson

(1865) described a 30 year old lady with lesions suggestive of lupus vulgaris on the face, causing severe disfigurement. Tilbury Fox, 1870 felt that "Lupus" which means wolf is called so "from the ulcerating and devouring character of the disease and regarded it as a "scrofulous inflammation and ulceration". The postmortem wart which was noted in medical personnel and butchers doing autopsies on cadavers infected with tuberculosis, developing warty lesions on the fingers was first proved to be tuberculous in 1884 and it was termed verruca necrogenica by Wilks, in 1886.

Rokitansky and Virchow successfully transmitted this disease to experimental animals and described the histopathological characteristics in great detail. Freidlander demonstrated the great similarity in histopathology of lupus vulgaris and tuberculosis of other organs.

French investigators, mindful of the beneficial action of sunshine used vitamin 'D' and found useful in some forms of tuberculosis. This train led Charpy (1943) to use calciferol in a series of patients with lupus vulgaris. Dowling and Thomas (1944) independently treated cutaneous tuberculosis with calciferol. Feldman and Hinshaw (1944) investigated the use of streptomycin in tuberculosis and later in cutaneous tuberculosis. Dowling and Weddington, Russel and Thorne reported the progress of patients treated with INAH.[7]

Despite the enormous amount of research that has been done since Koch first isolated the etiological agent in 1882 knowledge about the pathogenesis of tuberculosis is still very incomplete.

Cutaneous tuberculosis is reported from all over the world. But the incidence is on the decline in the indigenous populations of Western Europe and USA, which parallels the decline in pulmonary tuberculosis. Such a trend is also seen in India, from 2% reported earlier [8 - 10]

Nevertheless, cutaneous tuberculosis remains a disease of importance, more so, as it can be effectively treated and eventually eradicated. The emerging danger however, is with the increasing prevalence of HIV infection and migrant populations leading to a likely upward trend in the incidence of cutaneous tuberculosis.

The word "tuberculosis" was probably first suggested by Schonlein in 1839. It was applied generically to all the manifestations of Phthisis, as the 'tubercle' is the fundamental anatomic basis of the disease.4 Older epithets were "phthisis" and "consumption", which referred to the marked wasting, characteristic of advanced disease. The lung is the most frequently affected organ but the disease has been termed "Morbus Percorpus", stressing that it may involve virtually any organ or system in the body [1]. The transmissible nature of tuberculosis was convincingly demonstrated by Villemin in 1868. In March 1882, Robert Koch isolated the tubercle bacillus in pure culture and established the well known Koch's postulates in the etiology of an infectious disease.

The incidence of tuberculosis is declining in most parts of the world on account of the availability of effective anti-tuberculous drugs, elimination of infected milk herds and general improvement in the living standards. However, tuberculosis continues to be a major public health problem in a developing countries due to many factors like, ignorance, illiteracy, poverty and malnourishment. Though not a significant health hazard, cutaneous tuberculosis is not uncommon.

After Rene-Theophile-Hyacinthe Laennec's earliest description of his own prosector's wart in 1826, cutaneous tuberculosis has been described in an astonishing variety of clinical expressions [11] The chronic, infectious, world-wide disease tuberculosis is caused by several species of *mycobacteria*, collectively designated as the tubercle bacilli [12]. Some workers use the term tubercle bacilli, synonymously with *Mycobacterium tuberculosis* [1]. The generic name *Mycobacterium* which means 'fungus-bacterium' was given in 1896, by Lehmann and Neumann, to a group of bacteria, which produce the characteristic mould like pellicle , when grown on liquid media.

At the beginning of this century, *M.tuberculosis* was the only species of *Mycobacterium* associated with and isolated from human disease. Other species of *Mycobacteria* were categorized as non-tuberculous mycobacteria, atypical, MOTT (mycobacteria other than tubercle bacilli), opportunistic, environmental, NTNLM (non-tuberculous, non- leprous mycobacteria). Runyon (1959) classified *Mycobacteria* by their ability to produce a yellow pigment (a carotenoid) and by their rate of growth. The *mycobacteria* of dermatological interest include *M. marinum, M. kansasi, M. scrofulaceum, M .szulgei, M.tuberculosis, M. avium, M. ulcerans, M. smegmatis, M.chelonei, M.fortuitum and M. leprae.* Now, more than 71 recognized species of *mycobacteria* are described [13] (Shinnick and Good, 1994). In recent times, *atypical mycobacteria* are broadly grouped into pathogens and non-pathogens, with the understanding that non-pathogens rarely become pathogens [14].

Morphology of Mycobacterium Tuberculosis

Mycobacterium tuberculosis (M.tuberculosis) belongs to the genus *Mycobacterium*, family *Mycobacteriaceae*, and order *Actinomycetales.* [13] They are facultative, intracellular parasites. [15] They are slender, straight or slightly curved, 3.0μ × 0.3μ, strictly aerobic, non-motile, non- sporing, rods with a waxy coating, that makes them resistant to most stains. The bacilli are slow growing, weakly gram - positive, showing "acid-fastness" ('red-snappers'), when stained by the Ziehl-Neelsen method. Acid-fastness is thought to be due to the trapped Fuchsin-mycolate complex in the uniquely thick cell wall [16]. The cell wall is composed of an interlacing layer of lipids, peptidoglycans and arabinomannans and gives the *mycobacteria,* another useful characteristic of their resistance to the lethal effects of acids, alkalis and detergents[17].

Ordinary laboratory media do not support growth of *mycobacteria* and special substances such as egg, potato, blood or albumin are necessary as enrichment.15. When cultured *in vitro*, colonies are opaque, dry, and off-white to cream-colored, with a nodular or wrinkled surface and irregular edges. Optimal growth temperature is 37° C and multiplication does not occur, both at 25° C or 45°C. Growth of *mycobacteria* is 20 -100 times slower than that of other bacteria. Hence it takes 4 - 6 weeks to obtain a colony of *M.tuberculosis*, for identification or drug sensitivity studies [18 – 19]

Mycobacterium has no known exotoxins, endotoxins or histiolytic enzymes. Its pathogenecity is related to its ability to escape killing by macrophages and induce delayed hypersensitivity (DH).

Mycobacterial Properties of Relevance to Human Disease [1]

The mycobacterial cell wall is the most complex of all in nature. It consists of four main layers.

1. The first, innermost layer is composed of murein or peptidoglycan- a substance found with minor variations in all bacteria. It consists of long polysaccharide chains, cross linked by shorter penta peptide chains, thereby forming a huge netlike macromolecule which gives the bacterial cell its shape and rigidity. In addition, the murein layer is responsible for the adjuvant activity of mycobacteria. Purified peptidoglycan induces granuloma formation in experimental animals.1
2. The next layer is composed of arabinogalactan, a branched polysacharide containing arabinose and galactose and also forming a net like macromolecule. Attached to this structure are long-chain fatty acids termed mycolic acids.
3. These mycolic acids contain about 80 carbon atoms, 60 or so in a long chain and about 20 in a shorter branch. These fatty acids form the third layer- a dense pallisade which gives the cell its thickness, high lipid content and hydrophobic nature. The mycolic acids are responsible for the acid-fastness, and their synthesis is the target of INAH.
4. The fourth and the outermost layer contain a complex group of substances collectively termed mycosides and contain peptides, sugars, and lipids. They are analogous to the O antigens of the Gram negative enteric bacteria.

Mycosides are responsible for colony morphology, agglutination serotypes and in some cases, virulence. They are thought to contribute to the electron- transparent capsule-like structure surrounding some species of mycobacteria within the macrophages and therefore have a protective function.

Other superficially situated sugar-containing lipids include the following:

"Cord factor" or surface glycolipid (trehalose-6, 6'- dimycolate) causes the bacilli to orient themselves parallel to one another, so that growth occurs in the form of serpentine cords (Wolinsky,1994) *in vitro*.18 Virulent strains have cord factors on their surface, whereas, avirulent strains do not . Injection of purified cord factor into mice produces the characteristic granuloma [19].

1. Sulfatides / Sulfolipids: are surface glycolipids containing sulfur that are present on virulent strains. They prevent the fusion of phagosomes of macrophages containing *M.tuberculosis*, with the lysosomes. Sulfatides help the *M.tuberculosis* to scavenge the potent microbicidal molecules like reactive oxygen and nitrogen intermediaries [20].
2. Lipoarabinomannan (LAM) – A major hetero polysaccharide similar in structure to the endotoxin of gram negative bacteria. The cell wall LAM constitutes 0.5% of mycobacterial weight [21]. Biological activities of LAM include

A. Strong seroreactivity,
B. Inhibition of IFN-γ mediated activation of macrophages,
C. Induction of cytokine production and release by macrophages,
D. Scavenging reactive oxygen intermediaries (ROI),
E. Suppression of T cell proliferation.

The effect of LAM on induction of TGF β appears to be dominant over induction by the pro-inflammatory cytokines i.e., TNFα, TNFβ, IL-1, IL-6, and IL-10 [22]. It inhibits macrophage activation by interferon gamma (IFNγ). It also induces macrophages to secrete interleukin (IL-10) and tumor necrosis factor alpha (TNFα) or cachectin. TNF-α causes fever, weight loss and tissue damage, while IL-10 suppresses T-cell proliferation induced by *mycobacteria.*19 *M.tuberculosis* is well equipped to scavenge potent microbicidal molecules by moieties like cell wall LAM and sulfatides [20].

In addition to the mycosides and polysacharide antigens, Mycobacteria contain many soluble antigens. These antigens include most cytoplasmic and secreted proteins and soluble carbohydrates and are divided into four groups [13].

Group I antigens are common to all species of *mycobacterium* and some may also be found in species of *nocardia* and *corynebacterium.*

Group II antigens are found in only slow growing *mycobacterium* species.

Group III antigens are found in rapidly growing species of *Mycobacterium* and also in species of *Nocardia.*

Group IV antigens are those unique to an individual species.

Overall, these groupings suggest that *mycobacteria* evolved from a common ancestral form and that rapid and slow growers diverged early in evolution. The sharing of antigens by the various species probably accounts for the lack of specificity of serological tests for tuberculosis. By various immunochemical and immunoelectrophoretic techniques, up to 90 distinct antigens are identified [13].

Tuberculosis in humans is caused by Mycobacterium *tuberculosis, M.bovis* and under certain conditions, the *Bacillus Calmette Guerin* (BCG), the attenuated strain of *M.bovis,* may also be responsible.23 There is however, strong evidence that these, together with a group of strains termed *M. africanum* are no more than variants of a single species.24 *M.africanum* is a rather heterogenous group of strains isolated originally from man in Equatorial Africa, which appear to bridge the gap between the human and bovine bacilli [1].

Phylogenetic trees of the genus *Mycobacterium* have been constructed and all recognized species of *Mycobacterium* are closely related to each other and distantly related to members of the other genera [13].

Pathogenesis and History of the Evolution of the Disease

Human disease is usually spread by droplets and hence the portal of entry is often the lung, but may also be the tonsils, intestine or rarely the skin or mucous membranes. It is estimated that a patient with positive sputum can infect an average of 10 other persons [25]. In a *Mycobacterium tuberculosis* naïve individual, subsequent to an aerosol infection, with a few (up to 5 bacilli) a primary focus of infection is established [26]. The organism is transmitted through inhalation, ingestion, or inoculation [27].

The common route of infection is the respiratory tract, by droplets spread while speaking, coughing, sneezing and singing. The droplets are of 1-5 microns and when they are inhaled by susceptible (tuberculin negative) persons, they may be deposited in the alveoli. Spread takes place rapidly via the lymphatics to the lymphnodes draining the area. The granuloma that forms at the site of pulmonary infection constitutes the Ghon's focus; and this together with the enlarged hilar nodes, is the primary complex of Ranke [1].

Some of the organisms by haematogenous spread reach finally the apices of the lung, where the Po2 is particularly high, and lie dormant there. (Simon's focus). Other organs that have rich arterial supplies, such as brain, kidneys, and the ends of growing long bones also may similarly be involved. In about 4-6 weeks, the T cell mediated immunity is activated and the tuberculin test becomes positive. In only 5% of the newly infected, the infection progresses to disease in a few weeks or months.

The primary lesion presumably develops at the site of implantation by a single airborne particle bearing one or a few bacilli.28 In the lung, Ghon's focus may be absorbed, become fibrotic and calcified, or breakdown, liquefy and discharge bacilli into the lung.

The subsequent course depends on virulence of the bacilli and immunological responses of the host. Often the organisms fail to thrive and the disease is arrested; less often it becomes progressive. Sometimes the organisms may remain dormant after a primary infection, only to reactivate later causing a recrudescence of the primary infection.

On the skin, the primary focus is a tuberculous chancre, and if the regional lymphnodes breakdown, scrofuloderma occurs [25].

Primary infection may also occur via the intestine with the involvement of the mesenteric lymph nodes or via the tonsils with secondary cervical adenitis; such alimentary tract infection results usually from the ingestion of milk infected with *M. bovis*, but sometimes from the use of eating utensils or ingestion of food contaminated with *M.tuberculosis* [28]. The reaction of human tissues to tubercle bacilli occurs in a sequence. Initially, an acute non-specific inflammatory reaction takes place, when bacilli multiply, but cannot be phagocytosed and killed by the neutrophil polymorphs. By about 3-6 weeks, the characteristic tubercle forms.

T lymphocytes interact with mycobacterial antigens displayed on the surface of antigen presenting cells (APC) and release lymphokines, interleukins and interferons. These are then responsible for the activation, and expression of MHC class II antigens and IL-2R on the T-lymphocytes. There is accumulation of macrophages in 14 days. Macrophages then phagocytose the organisms, but their efficacy in killing them crucially depends on enhanced activation. The macrophages in all chronic granulomatous diseases in man are activated by lymphokines, particularly by γ-IFN, and also by a positive feedback loop involving 1,25(OH)2 chole calciferol (calcitriol), which is formed from circulating 25(OH) vitamin D3 by IFN-γ activated macrophages. Leakage of this calcitriol from the lesions into the systemic circulation accounts for the subtle alterations in the calcium metabolism, which can occur in this condition. In view of the role of calcitriol, vitamin D was used successfully for the treatment of lupus vulgaris in 1940s, but had detrimental effects on TB in deep sites [29]. T-Cell allergy to tuberculous antigens induces secretion of cytokines that recruit and activate macrophages.

The monocytes enlarge, their nucleus becomes eccentric and, their cytoplasm more abundant, and they tend to aggregate first into loose sheets of cells and then more tightly into spherical aggregates or granulomas. The cells comprisng these granulomas develop eccentric vesicular nuclei and abundant pale cytoplasm. Although the cells remain initially distinct, later their cytoplasm borders become indistinct when viewed under the light microscope. Under electron microscope, this is seen to be due to the close interlocking of the pseudopodia of the neighboring cells. These characteristic mononuclear cells are called epithelioid cells, because they are closely packed like epithelial cells without interposed connective tissue. They are not joined by functional complexes, do not closely resemble epithelium morphologically and are the progeny of monocytes and not epithelium [30].

Epithelioid cells are characterized by their well-developed granular endoplasmic reticulum, numerous lysosomes and high levels of lysosomal enzyme activity. They are less actively phagocytic than typical macrophages. They are considered as macrophages specialized for secretory functions and for degradation and destruction of microbes.

A few epithelioid cells fuse to form the Langhans' type of giant cells. Within 30 days, as delayed hypersensitivity increases, there is caseation necrosis within the granuloma. This caseation, termed so because of the dry crumbly appearance like cheese is probably mediated by the cytokines like TNF and the macrophage proteases. The necrotic process kills many mycobacteria in the lesion, but they are not eliminated [31 – 32]. Memory T cells generated during initial sensitization remain in circulation and in lymphoid organs for a long time [25]

The granuloma can follow several possible courses. The number of organisms may decrease, a fibrous capsule may form in the surrounding zone, and calcium salts may get deposited in the caseous material. Sometimes the calcium is deposited in concentric laminations known as Liesegang rings [30].

The necrotic granuloma is typical of tuberculosis and other mycobacterial infections, but is not specific and is seen in many other infections involving this type of cell-mediated immunity like leishmaniasis, syphilis and histoplasmosis [33].

Sehgal et al. (1988) opined that, unlike in peripheral blood, CD4 T- lymphocytes predominate in the granuloma of lupus vulgaris and TBVC, while CD8 T-lymphocytes are more in scrofuloderma. The CD4/CD8 ratio also progressively decreases from lupus vulgaris to scrofuloderma, through TBVC. It is postulated that in cutaneous tuberculosis, the infection is compartmentalised and immunological upheavals operate locally. So, systemic effects are maintained at a minimum, while the immune response is enhanced at the site of infection.34

There are 3 strategies, by which mycobacteria survive within macrophages,

First, by poorly understood mechanisms, they inhibit fusion of the phagosome to the lysosomes.

Second, they neutralize reactive oxygen intermediates (ROI) by means of cell wall lipids including peptidoglycolipids and LAM, and by secreting the enzyme Superoxide dismutase.

Third, they escape from the phagosome and replicate in the cytoplasm of the cell [1].

The outcome of infection is dictated by a number of independent but interrelated factors, namely:

1. Immune status (CMI) of the host as a consequence of sensitization.
2. Route of infection
3. Pathogenicity / virulence of the infecting mycobacterial strain. (*M.tuberculosis* is the most virulent among all other *mycobacteria.)*
4. Size of the inoculum.

If CMI is impaired, the T-cell / macrophage system will not operate to contain the infection. The resulting pathology is less granulomatous with fewer activated macrophages and hence has a higher number of *mycobacteria.*

Classification of Skin Tuberculosis

Infection of the skin and subcutis by *M.tuberculosis* occurs by three routes i.e. direct inoculation into the skin, hematogenous spread from an internal focus and by direct extension (contiguity), from an underlying focus.

No entirely satisfactory classification exists. Darier (1896) separated proven tuberculous lesions from the remainder i.e., the tuberculides. Pillsbury, Shelly and Kligman, (1956) wrote that "in the skin , tuberculosis presents in an astonishing variety of forms, which have given rise to an unwieldy overextended number of descriptive terms and bewildering classification."

Cutaneous tuberculosis may be primary or secondary. Primary infection implies the absence of previous infection and must be subdivided into localized and hematogenous type. Secondary tuberculous skin infections develop in individuals who, having suffered a primary tuberculous infection and healed, are again exposed to infection. Beyt al. et al. (1980) [36], classified cutaneous tuberculosis based on suspected pathogenesis of the disease, clinical presentation, and histological evaluation. However, many cases clinically do not fit into this clinical and histological classification [35].

The classification proposed by Beyt et al. (1980) [36], and modified by Savin and Wilkinson (1986) [37], is as follows:

Inoculation Tuberculosis (Exogenous Source)

Tuberculous chancre
Warty tuberculosis
Lupus vulgaris (some)

Secondary Tuberculosis (Endogenous Source)

Contiguous Spread

Scrofuloderma

Auto Inoculation

Orificial tuberculosis

Hematogenous Tuberculosis

Acute miliary tuberculosis
Lupus vulgaris (some)
Tuberculous gumma

Eruptive Tuberculosis (Tuberculides)

Lichen scrofulosorum
Papular or papulonecrotic tuberculides
The synonymous terms for the different types of cutaneous tuberculosis are,

1. Tuberculous chancre

Primary inoculation
Tuberculous primary complex
Primary inoculation tuberculosis
Primary cutaneous tuberculosis

2. Warty Tuberculosis

Tuberculosis verrucosa cutis
Tuberculosis cutis verrucosa
Lupus verrucosus
Verruca necrogenica
Prosector's wart
Butcher's wart
Post-mortem wart
Anatomist's wart

3. Lupus Vulgaris

Tuberculosis luposa cutis
Tuberculosis luposa.

4. Acute Miliary Tuberculosis of the Skin

Acute disseminated miliary tuberculosis
Tuberculosis cutis miliaris disseminata
Tuberculosis cutis acuta genralisata
Tuberculosis miliaris generalisata

5. Tuberculous gumma

Metastatic tuberculous abscess
Gummatous tuberculosis
Tuberculosis colliquativa

6. Orificial Tuberculosis

Tuberculosis cutis orificialis
Tuberculosis ulcerosa cutis et mucosae
Tuberculosis orificialis

7. Scrofuloderma

Tuberculosis colliquativa cutis
Tuberculosis cutis colliquativa

Tuberculides

Tuberculides represent allergic reaction to showers of antigen reaching highly immune skin by hematogenous spread, from an internal focus. The tuberculous focus is not often clinically active at the time of eruption and the patient is usually in excellent health.

In case of facultative tuberculides, like nodular vasculitis and erythema nodosum, TB is one of the possible causes and is not the most common [35]. The tuberculides were detailed by Wolff and Tappeiner (1987) [23], under their respective headings and not under tuberculosis.

Primary Cutaneous Tuberculosis

It is a primary infection in an individual previously free of tuberculosis in any form. The disease is rare and occurs in infants [38], or in individuals whose occupation causes them to be exposed [39]. There is no previous exposure and no specific immunity to the *M.tuberculosis* bacilli at the time of inoculation. In such patients there is a recent documented tuberculin conversion [40].

Numerous reports have appeared describing inoculation TB since the time of Laennec (1826). Tscherning (1888), mentions a servant of a tuberculous master who wounded himself on a sputum cup, and developed tuberculosis. Chancellor (1914), described tuberculosis of the cheek, which was traced to the playful bite of a nurse. Other cases were reported after mouth to mouth resuscitation [41].

The primary cutaneous complex consists of the chancre together with regional lymphadenopathy. It is analogous to pulmonary Ghon's complex [42]. A chancre is an ulcerated nodule with ragged undermined edges that occurs at the site of earlier skin trauma and provides the portal of initial entry for the bacilli. Bacilli are numerous, in both the ulcer and its satellite lymphnodes. It is usually found on the limbs and rarely on the genitalia and anal region. Systemic symptoms are minimal or absent.

Inoculation tuberculosis accounts for only 5% of total primary tuberculosis [41 – 42]. Since *M. tuberculosis* is not capable of penetrating intact human skin, some sort of injury must be present for an infection to be established. Portals of entry often include such minor injuries as abrasions, puncture wounds, hangnails, and pyodermas. It affects children more commonly, with the face and exposed extremities being sites of predilection. Tuberculous chancres have also been reported after ritual circumcision, cardiopulmonary resuscitation, tattoos, inoculations and injections for immunization or therapy, ear piercing, venipuncture, misinoculation of laboratory animals, and sexual intercourse. Inoculation can also occur in the mucous membranes of the oral cavity after tooth extraction, in the tonsils from ingesting non-pasteurized milk, or in the ocular conjunctiva during ocular surgery [39 – 40]. Primary inoculation tuberculosis has been reported following a needle stick injury from a patient with AIDS and undiagnosed tuberculosis [43].

Clinical Features: After an incubation period of 3 to 4 weeks following inoculation, a small inflammatory papule develops, which quickly breaks down into an indolent, firm, non-tender, sharply delimited ulcer with no tendency for spontaneous healing for several weeks. After 3 to 8 weeks, tubercle bacilli reach the regional nodes, producing painless lymphadenitis. This ulceroglandular complex is the prototype of primary inoculation tuberculosis, the skin analog to the primary pulmonary Ghon complex.

Laboratory findings: Initially the tuberculin test is negative. The PPD usually becomes positive following the development of lymphadenopathy, although early treatment may prevent conversion.

Histopathology: primary inoculation tuberculosis in early stages shows acute neutrophilic reaction, with necrosis, ulceration and large number of tubercle bacilli. With the development of immunity in 3-6 weeks the lesion turns into a granuloma, characterized by epithelioid cells, Langhans' type of giant cells surrounded by a peripheral rim of lymphocytes. This is followed by development of caseous necrosis with subsequent decrease in bacterial load. Similar changes are also seen in lymph nodes.

Differential Diagnosis: Coccidiodomycosis, blastomycosis, syphilitic chancre and skin malignancy may resemble primary cutaneous tuberculosis [12]. The diagnosis is confirmed by the demonstration of the organisms with Ziehl- Nielsen's stain, culture and animal inoculation.

Course and Prognosis: The primary lesion heals by scarring usually in 1-3 weeks, though occasionally it may last up to one year. In patients with low immunity, in presence of heavy bacillary load miliary tuberculosis, which may prove fatal, occurs. Satisfactory host immunity with high degree of tuberculin sensitivity usually results. Latent foci may be locally activated or organisms may be shed into blood stream resulting in hematogenous dissemination to distant sites. By this mechanism lupus vulgaris or tuberculosis verrucosa cutis may develop as late complications of primary inoculation tuberculosis. As the lymphnodes liquefy, scrofuloderma may occur. Development of erythema nodosum as a nonspecific hypersensitivity reaction may also occur.

Scrofuloderma (Tuberculosis Cutis Colliquativa) [Plate: I]

Tuberculous lymphadenitis of the neck is also known as scrofula.1 It is probably derived from the latin word *Scrofa* - a brood sow , from the likeness of the cluster of nodes to piglets feeding from the sow. Others believe that it reflects the somewhat sow like features imparted to the victims by the swelling of the face and neck and the associated anemia.

Clinical features: Scrofuloderma involves the skin secondarily by extension from tuberculous lymph nodes, bones or joints. So, nodules occur on lymph nodes of the neck, sternal region, knees or ankles .The site of the first enlargement gives a clue to the place of origin of infection, for the path of lymphatic drainage is precise [44 – 45]. The swelling may seem to be confined to one group of nodes or may continue to others in the line of lymph flow. The onset of tuberculous lymphadenitis is usually slow and painless but can, in highly tuberculin sensitive persons, be acute with pyrexia and perinodal reaction. Whatever be the mode of onset, the glands usually become caseous44 although this softening may not happen for a considerable time, perhaps after an intercurrent infective illness.

The lymph nodes are initially firm, but caseation occurs and they become fluctuant resulting in draining sinuses, which discharge infectious purulent matter. These ulcerated or fistualized lesions become confluent and healing occurs by hypertrophic or cord like cicatrices. A swollen, distorted mass is created which eventually shows special patterns of scarring (tags, tongues and 'basket-handle' or 'bridge' scars), which look like miniature tube-grafts.46 Occasionally they appear to settle completely and calcify, but there is always the risk of enlargement and softening even after decades [44 - 45].

In earlier times, scrofuloderma was common in children—80% following an oral or tonsillar primary inoculation of bovine tuberculosis from infected milk [23 ,46]. Elderly individuals are also susceptible when their immunity is low. True tuberculous lymphadenitis is becoming less common in children and is more often due to atypical mycobacteria: *M avium*, *M intracellulare*, or *M scrofulaceum* [37]. Scrofuloderma occurs rarely from the introduction of exogenous tubercle bacilli into the subcutis by trauma, or by injections into individuals with previous latent or manifest tuberculosis. Scrofuloderma was described in a broad age range, from 18 months to 66 years [47].

Laboratory findings: Patients developing scrofuloderma have a weakened cell-mediated immunity overall but often maintain a positive PPD [34].

Histopathology: Tuberculous granulomas with massive caseous necrosis are seen in lower dermis at the margins of ulcers or abscesses. Epithelioid cells are seen in large numbers along with Langhans' giant cells. Acid-fast bacilli can be demonstrated in the lesions.

Lesions of sporotrichosis, actinomycosis, and pyogenic lymphadenitis may show similar clinical aspects [12].

Course and Prognosis: Scrofuloderma is usually associated with tuberculosis else where in the body, usually lungs or abdomen. Occurrence of lupus vulgaris in the vicinity or in the scar of lesions of scrofuloderma and malignant lesions like an epithelioma is also reported. Rarely systemic amyloidosis also can occur in scrofuloderma.

Tuberculosis Cutis Verrucosa (Tbvc) [Plate: II]

Tuberculosis of the skin arising from the direct inoculation of a tuberculin–sensitive individual (TBVC), is a rare disease [48].

Originally termed verruca necrogenica by Wilks and Poland in 1862, a variety of descriptive terms have been employed, including prosector's wart, postmortem wart, anatomical tubercle, cadaver wart, anatomic wart and warty tuberculosis. In the past, the disease was usually found among pathologists, autopsy room attendants, butchers and undertakers. Advances in the chemotherapy of tuberculosis and improvements in sanitation and hygiene have made these lesions increasingly rare in modern times [48]. Laennec, in 1826, published what was probably the first description of prosector's wart, based on his own disease contracted in the autopsy room. Sir William Osler (1889) wrote of his experiences with "the Anatomical tubercle" in the Montreal Medical journal; where he described 8-10 scars from these warts, which he had at times on his hands during the past 15 years. Sir Osler used oleate of mercury to treat the warty lesions, while Laennec had employed butter of antimony (antimony trichloride), earlier in the century, as a local remedy for his dermal lesions [45].

Most cases are due to an exogenous reinfection in individuals with marked cutaneous hypersensitivity and good immunity. Rarely, auto-inoculation from sputum may cause the lesions. Adult men are most commonly affected [12]. Warty tuberculosis was the most prevalent form of cutaneous tuberculosis in Hong Kong, where it was reported predominantly in children [49].

Clinical Features: The lesions start as indurated and keratotic plaques, closely simulating verruca vulgaris. Small warty papules gradually increase in number and then coalesce to form round or oval, verrucous, red brown plaques. The surface has fissures and clefts and a bead of pus can be expressed from them. Usually one or two lesions are present. The verrucous lesions are located mostly on the dorsal surfaces of feet, hands, wrists, knees and sometimes, the buttocks. In adults, they are more common on hands; in children on legs [49]. The lesions have been frequently reported on the hands in Europe and on the lower limbs in the Eastern countries [50]. They may heal spontaneously over years, leaving atrophic scars. Generally, lymphadenopathy is not associated, although it has been reported [35, 51]. The asymptomatic lesions occur at sites of trauma. Partly due to the immunological background and partly due to specific terrain of the acral skin, there is a strong tendency to verrucous hyperplasia and to fibrosis in these lesions [53].

Some of the documented unusual clinical presentations of tuberculosis verrucosa cutis are perianal ulcerations from gastrointestinal inoculation, sclerotic masses, fungating granulomas, disseminated tuberculosis with cutaneous and pulmonary involvement in an immunocompetent patient, and multifocal guttate tuberculosis verrucosa cutis [40].

Laboratory Findings: These patients have moderate to good immunity and PPD test is positive.

Histopathology: Hyperkeratosis, hypergranulosis, acanthosis, and papillomatosis of the epidermis are present in tuberculosis verrucosa cutis. Variable numbers of tuberculoid granulomas with a modest amount of caseous necrosis and a few acid-fast bacilli are seen in the mid-dermis. With time, marked fibrosis occurs.

This type of cutaneous tuberculosis must be distinguished from cases of chromomycosis.12

Course and Prognosis: Lesions may evolve and last for a period of years or even decades. Prognosis is usually good.

Lupus Vulgaris (Lv) [Plate: III]

An ulceration that tore into the flesh like the ravages of a wolf probably fitted the clinical description and explains the word “lupus”, which means wolf. The commonness of this condition in earlier times accounts for the adjective vulgaris, in lupus vulgaris.46 The earliest description of LV was by Erasmus Wilson in 1865 [49].

Lupus vulgaris occurs in individuals with immunity produced by previous tuberculous infection. As many as two thirds of patients with lupus vulgaris are found to have visceral foci of tuberculosis. Of these, 40% have tuberculous adenitis or involvement of the mucous membranes, and 10% to 20% have pulmonary, bone, or joint tuberculosis [40].

Children are most commonly affected. The state of allergy and the degree of immunity are closely related to the morphologic manifestations in cutaneous tuberculosis . For this reason, lupus vulgaris is in most instances a chronic slowly progressive disease, beginning as a small lupus nodule, growing peripherally and forming an ever enlarging plaque, the character of which changes when the inflammation brings about noticeable alterations in the epidermis or cutis. If the epidermis becomes hyperkeratotic, the lesion assumes a verrucous character, or if lymphatic stasis is pronounced in the corium, the lesion becomes tumefied, and so on, but the basic process is the same, a tuberculous inflammation beginning and extending in the cutis and having certain characteristics which are unique for lupus vulgaris [52].

The bacilli reach the skin from another active focus of tuberculosis through hematogenous route or by contiguity. The lesions occur commonly around the nose and on the cheeks in western countries. This localization could be due to the rich and porous venous plexuses with stasis, cold and hypoxia, and impaired fibrinolysis and host defense at a lower temperature.46 Though lesions may occur on the extremities, involvement of the trunk is rare. In India and many developing nations, the lower extremities, especially the buttocks, are the primary site of involvement. It is exceedingly rare for the mucous membranes to be involved. The initial lesions are usually solitary, though occasionally two or more lesions can occur.

Clinical Features: The individual lesions begin as reddish brown or blue papules that coalesce to form a plaque with a serpiginous border. The plaque grows by peripheral extension and healing at one end. The 'apple jelly' colored nodules is classically described at the periphery. They are small semi-translucent nodules, characterized by brownish red color and a soft consistency and represent cell-rich, and fiber free areas. A thin piece of glass slide pressed against the plaque (Diascopy test) may exhibit the diagnostic "apple jelly "color. Bacilli are sparse and rarely demonstrable, but guinea pig inoculation is confirmatory.

Laboratory features: Bacilli in lupus vulgaris are few and sparse. Inoculated guinea pigs usually succumb to disseminated tuberculosis at the anticipated time when inoculated with lesional tissue. Tuberculin testing is usually positive.

Histopathology: The lesions are characterized by epithelioid cell granulomas with Langhans' giant cells, mononuclear cells and peripheral rim of lymphocytes. Caseous necrosis is uncommon and minimal. Bacilli are difficult to demonstrate. Secondary epidermal changes like atrophy, ulceration, acanthosis and pseudoepitheliomatous hyperplasia may be seen. Development of squamous cell carcinoma also may be noticed.

The differential diagnosis must be made from cases of sporotrichosis, basal cell carcinoma and late syphilis.

Course and Prognosis: Lupus vulgaris is a chronic disfiguring disease may progress over years or even decades. The disease is usually present for about five years before definitive diagnosis is made. A case of a hospital employee who has had lesions for more than 20 years was reported from a rural teaching hospital in Cuddalore district. Multifocal lesions are also known to occur. Severe scarring resulting in severe mutilation and disfigurement of face with destruction of nose and distortion of mouth and scaly lesions resembling psoriasis were also reported in literature 54, 55 Occurrence of squamous cell carcinoma is known. Other tumors like basal cell carcinoma, Hodgkin lymphoma also may be rarely associated with Lupus vulgaris. Occurrence of tuberculides like Lichen scrofulosorum and papulonecrotic tuberculides in conjunction with Lupus vulgaris is known.

Tuberculosis Orificialis

These lesions occur at the mucocutaneous junctions of the nose, oral and anogenital areas, due to the auto-inoculation of *mycobacteria* from severe visceral tuberculosis. It is common in middle-aged or older persons. Men are more often affected.

Small yellowish or reddish nodule rapidly breaks down to form a painful, shallow ulcer with undermined bluish edges. The surrounding mucosa is swollen and the ulcer is covered by a pseudo-membranous material.

Large numbers of AFB can be detected in biopsy sections and culture confirms the diagnosis. The lesions should be differentiated from, aphthous ulcers, carcinoma and syphilitic lesions.

Tuberculosis Miliaris Generalisata (Disseminated Tuberculosis)

Tuberculosis miliaris generalisata occurs usually in infants or children with unmistakable signs of internal tuberculosis. It is caused by bacilli showered from an internal tuberculous focus to the skin. Tuberculin sensitivity is usually absent probably because of overwhelming infection.56

Minute erythematous macules or papules and purpuric lesions are disseminated to all parts of the body. Patients usually have acute miliary disease of the internal organs prior to hematogenous dissemination.

Tuberculides

A tuberculide is a cutaneous reaction to an extra cutaneous tuberculous infection. Used as a suffix, "-ides" indicate membership of a family or class. In Greek it would mean 'the son of '. In astronomy, the showers of meteors are also called 'ides'. If ides are considered as belonging to a family , they are rather like the poor relations or country cousins of the more sumptuous and well-established family members. They are apt to turn up having lost their papers and credentials [46].

Darier (1896), introduced the concept of tuberculides and they are classified as follows: [23,35,36].

True (Probable)Tuberculides

Lichen scrofulosorum
Papulonecrotic tuberculides

Facultative (Possible) Tuberculides

Erythema Induratum of Bazin
Erythema nodosum

Non-Tuberculides (Former Tuberculides)

Lupus miliaris disseminatus faciei
Rosacea-like tuberculides
Lichenoid tuberculides

Clinical Features

True (Probable) Tuberculides

1. Papulonecrotic Tuberculides [Plate: IV]

Pautrier first described this entity in 1936 and established its tuberculous etiology [57]. This condition is characterized by an eruption of necrotizing papules, occurring in successive symmetrical crops, particularly affecting the extremities and responding to antituberculous drugs. This disease affects mostly adults and children . Females outnumber males by a ratio of 3 : 1.58 The small symptomless nodules appear on the elbows, knees, buttocks and face. Involvement of the glans penis was also described [58]. They become necrotic in some weeks and are covered with a small, dark crust leaving a varioloid scar. The proposed etiology of the skin lesions is hematogenous spread of bacilli that causes an Arthus reaction and delayed hypersensitivity.58 Though *M.tuberculosis* is the most common etiological agent , Callahan (1997), recently reported a case of PNT reaction to *M. kansasi* [57].

Tuberculin sensitivity is intense. Biopsy, a general physical examination and tuberculin testing is necessary to establish the diagnosis. The histopathologic characteristics depend on the age of the lesions and range from sub-acute lymphocytic vasculitis to granulomatous vasculitis with focal infarction and coagulative necrosis, which is characteristically " flask shaped" , when viewed under low power.58(Wilson Jones, 1986).

The patients active immune systems destroy all evidence of the bacilli in the skin, making stains and cultures negative [59]. However PCR examination may reveal evidence of *M. tuberculosis* [60]. It should be distinguished from prurigo, vasculitis, insect bites and pityriasis lichenoides [12].

2. Lichen Scrofulosorum

Lichen scrofulosorum was first recognised by Hebra (1868). Miesher (1955), described the association of lichen scrofulosorum with tuberculosis of lymph nodes, bones and joints, although the infection was not always obvious at the time of development of the rash. Along with papulonecrotic tuberculides, lichen scrofulosorum is also considered a 'true tuberculide [35].

Lichen scrofulosorum type of tuberculides are rare. Groups of very small, non itching lichenoid papules, on the back and sides of the trunk characterize the condition. Patients have a marked tuberculin sensitivity. Most of the patients are children with visceral tuberculosis. The disappearance of the lesions and the improvement of internal disease with antituberculous treatment confirms the diagnosis. The disease is frequently overlooked as it is mistaken for keratosis pilaris and phrynoderma.

Histopathology of Tuberculides

Superficial dermal granulomas are seen in the histology sections. Caseation necrosis may or may not be present and histologically distinguishing this lesion from sarcoidosis may be impossible[35,47]. The granulomas may or may not be contiguous with hair follicles or sweat ducts. Bacilli are not found.

Facultative (Possible) Tuberculides

1. Erythema Induratum of Bazin

Erythema induratum was described by Bazin in 1861, and usually occurs in young women who have glandular tuberculosis and acrocyanosis. Males are almost never affected [61]. Also called nodular vasculitis, its true association with tuberculosis was doubted [62].owever, since patients with erythema induratum have intense tuberculin sensitivity, and recover with antituberculous treatment, it was accepted to be a true tuberculide. Mycobacterial DNA rated in the lesions by PCR technique [60].

The lower calf is often affected. The initial lesions are firm blue-red, painful nodules persisting for three or four months. They occur in crops of painful 1-2 cm nodules, usually on the posterolateral calves [47, 62]. Lesions have also been described on the arms, thighs, feet and buttocks. They tend to dry up and heal and then recur. In course of months, some central softening is noted in the overlying skin and it progresses to ulcers. The ulcers are deeply excavated, with undermined edges and are irregular in shape.

Histopathology

Nodular vasculitis describes the histology of this condition. Arteritis, lobular panniculitis, and fat necrosis are the diagnostic features [63]. Bacilli cannot be demonstrated by Z-N stain, though recently *M.tuberculosis* DNA could be demonstrated by PCR analysis [64].

Much controversy appears in the literature regarding EIB and its status as a tuberculid.64 Arguments against are:

1. Inability to culture AFB from lesional biopsy specimens , thereby violating Koch's postulates;
2. The high incidence of TB in the normal population, producing a coincidental but not causal relation between the two;
3. The variability of PPD results;
4. The inconsistent reponse to ATT, and
5. The positive response to systemic steroids.

Arguments supporting the association of EIB with a tuberculous origin include;

1. The hyperresponsiveness to PPD in most patients [62].
2. Marked clinical reponse to adequate ATT
3. The T-Cell hyperresponsiveness of patients specifically to PPD
4. Low amounts of tuberculous DNA in lesions by PCR [60].

2. Erythema Nodosum

Erythema nodosum clinically resembles erythema induratum in that, it causes tender, red nodules, usually on the legs of women. However, the lesions occur more commonly on the anterior legs and rarely ulcerate. Erythema nodosum can be associated rarely with tuberculosis and more commonly with other infectious conditions, sarcoidosis and drugs.

Histopathology

Erythema nodosum is a septal panniculitis. Early lesions may have neutrophils in the fat septa; older lesions have lymphohistiocytic infiltrates. Histologically, erythema nodosum can be distinguished from erythema induratum by the absence of significant lobular infiltrates, vasculitis, and necrosis [63].

Nodular allergic vasculitis, gummatous syphilis and the nodose lesions caused by iodides and bromides should be distinguished from erythema nodosum and EIB.

Diagnosis of Cutaneous Tuberculosis

Diagnosis is based on 6 relative and 2 absolute criteria, apart from other supportive immunological evidence [35].

Relative Criteria

The clinical history and signs
Presence of active, proven tuberculosis elsewhere in the body
Histopathology
Presence of acid fast bacilli in the lesion.
Positive tuberculin test.
Effect of specific anti-tuberculous therapy

Absolute Criteria

Culture of *M.tuberculosis* organisms on Lowenstein – Jensen's medium. Growth occurs in 4-6 weeks.

Recovery of tubercle bacilli from animal inoculation using guinea pigs.

Gurmohan Singh, (1994)61 held that when a lesion develops at a site of trauma and persists in the face of antibiotic therapy for a long time; suspicion must arise of a mycobacterial etiology.

Mantoux Test

The tuberculin test is a means of identification of the infection before it produces active disease [65]. Mx test indicates the cell-mediated hypersensitivity of the skin to tuberculin. The response is higher in re-infection when compared to reactivation tuberculosis. This *in vivo* test correlates well with the migratory index (MI) of lymphocytes to tuberculin antigen, assayed through lymphocyte migration inhibition test (LMIT)[67]

Mantoux test has limited diagnostic application in countries where BCG vaccination is part of routine immunization programme. A majority of adults are tuberculin positive.

Only a negative tuberculin test is useful, as the positive reaction indicates an infection and not disease. CDC guidelines (1990), for the interpretation of skin test results are shown in table 1.

As per the CDC recommendations [68] (1997) HIV infected persons with positive PPD tuberculin test should be evaluated to exclude active TB and given preventive INAH therapy, if indicated which is effective in reducing the incidence of active TB among patients with HIV infection and latent TB. However, HIV+ve patients may be PPD –ve, because of cutaneous anergy.

Differential Diagnosis

The histological signature of the tubercle bacillus is susceptible to forgery [69]. The typical features are characteristic but the variations are many, especially if caseation necrosis is absent or the subject's immunity is poor. Other mycobacterial infections cannot be differentiated except by culture at 25 0- 30 0C.

In sarcoidosis, all the features except caseation necrosis may be present and differentiation from lupus vulgaris may be impossible though the epithelioid cell foci tend to be more scattered and well defined and surrounded by relatively fewer lymphocytes and by reticulin.

In tuberculoid leprosy, a neural and perineural involvement is the only distinguishing feature.

In leishmaniasis, blastomycosis, and chromoblastomycosis, the causative organism clinches the diagnosis. In tertiary syphilis, there are more pronounced vascular changes and a plasma cell infiltrate.

Rosacea and panniculitis may cause confusion due to the presence of a non-specific tuberculoid inflammatory infiltrate, with irregular groups of epithelioid cells. Typical tubercle formation is absent.

Limitations for the Diagnosis of Cutaneous Tuberculosis

The demonstration of bacilli is not easy by the usual procedures i.e. smears, culture, and guinea pig inoculations. The recovery of bacilli in smears or histological preparations gives a presumptive diagnosis. Guinea pig inoculation provides the absolute proof of pathogenicity. Cultures separate *M.tuberculosis* bacilli from other *Mycobacteria*.

Active tuberculosis elsewhere in the body supports the diagnosis of tuberculides. Sometimes the diagnosis of cutaneous tuberculosis is made only by elimination of other diseases or by a therapeutic trial. If the lesions do not improve after 6 weeks treatment in adequate dose, it is unlikely to be tuberculosis.

The inherent limitations of conventional methods for the diagnosis of cutaneous tuberculosis are:

The smear examination for AFB is only presumptive evidence, with very low sensitivity to detect scant mycobacteria. in the cutaneous lesions.

The recovery of *mycobacteria* takes a long time i.e. 6-8 weeks.

Other specific, sensitive and rapid methods for the diagnosis are

1. Identification of mycobacterial antigens in tissues by radio immunoassay [70 – 71]
2. Enzyme linked immunosorbent assay (ELISA) for the detection of immunoglobulins to mycobacterial antigens [66,72]
3. Identification of Mycobacterial DNA by using DNA probes, either 125 I-labelled or acridium-ester labeled [73,74]. However, due to the low sensitivity, these techniques require a week-long amplification culture of the specimen, before assay.
4. Polymerase chain reaction (PCR) is an in vitro technique that enables the amplification of specific mycobacterial DNA sequences.

5. Recently, mtp 40 has been identified as a highly specific genomic fragment of *M. tuberculosis* 75 (Portillo, 1991) and may be used for identification, following amplification from tissue specimens without resorting to culture. It is a highly sensitive, specific and rapid method to identify *M. tuberculosis* and helps to differentiate from other *mycobacteria*.

Polymerase Chain Reaction (PCR)

DNA amplification by PCR is a rapid and sensitive method for detection of M.tuberculosis organisms in samples. Fewer than 10 microorganisms could be detected; however, precise estimation of the sensitivity is difficult [76]. PCR positivity was reported in cases of cutaneous tuberculosis even when organisms could not be demonstrated by Z.N. staining or and also by culture of skin biopsy specimens [77].

Two mycobacterial sequences have served as targets for amplification. They are the mycobacteria specific DNA sequences IS 6110, which is present as repeats within a genome and the gene coding the 65KDa heat shock protein which is expressed as an antigen in many mycobacteria (65 KDa antigen DNA).

The identification of the target sequence of the DNA does not imply organism viability. It might be possible to identify a DNA sequence specific for M. tuberculosis in samples where culture results are negative either because the organism is present in too few numbers to grow in culture or because host defenses had rendered the mycobacteria incapable of growing [76].

Treatment

Mycobacteria have a special characteristic that allows them to convert to an inactive metabolic state when environmental conditions become unsuitable for growth. Three treatable populations of tubercle bacilli have been postulated.

1. 1. The largest group, which grows extracellular, is liable to become resistant and is best treated by two bactericidal drugs.
2. 2. A much smaller group of intermittently or slowly growing organisms is found within the macrophages at an acid pH.
3. A third similar group exists in caseous areas with a neutral pH.

Rifampicin is bactericidal to all the three populations.

Isoniazid is bactericidal for both the actively growing bacilli in cavities and for those within the macrophages.

Streptomycin is bactericidal against rapidly growing extracellular bacilli.

Pyrazinamide is effective against intracellular organisms only.

All the other drugs are bacteriostatic [78].

First Line of Drugs

Isoniazid (INH)
Rifampicin (RMP)
Ethambutol (EMB)
Streptomycin (SM)

Second-Line Drugs

Pyrazinamide (PZA)
Ethionamide (ETH)
Cycloserine (CS)
Capreomycin (CM)
Viomycin (VM)
Para-aminosalicylic acid (PAS)

Most previous regimes used more than one antituberculous drug in different combinations for 12-24 months.

The treatment of cutaneous tuberculosis is the same as that for systemic tuberculosis [78 - 79]. With the advent of HIV pandemic, this is very important. The chemotherapy recommended by WHO has the advantage of achieving a high cure rate, reducing morbidity, preventing the emergence of resistant strains and eliminating the "persisters". A therapeutic response to anti tuberculous drugs also helps to confirm the diagnosis.

Well known antituberculous drugs, such as isoniazid (INH), rifampicin, ethambutol, and pyrazinamide are the drugs commonly used in the treatment of skin tuberculosis.

Table 1. CDC guidelines (1990), for the interpretation of skin test results.

Size of induration	situations considered as +ve result
<5mm	Never
5 / >5mm	Doubtful
10/ >10 mm	Persons with HIV infection ,Persons in contact with an infectious TB patient, HIV negative IV drug abusers and patients with risk of acquiring TB; persons born in countries with high prevalence of TB; persons from high risk communities; medically under served persons and residents of long term care facilities.
> 15 mm	All others

The American college of chest physicians (ACCP) recommends a 9 month course of INH, RMP, usually supplemented by a 2-3 months' initial phase of one additional drug, usually EMB or SM or PZA [79 - 80].

The ACCP recommendations are most relevant when the tuberculous skin infection is associated with pulmonary or extra-pulmonary focus of TB. These recommendations may have to be modified depending on the availability, cost, and resistance problems in developing countries.35

Drainage, debridement and surgical intervention may be required in cases of scrofuloderma, gumma, orificial TB, ocular and peri-ocular forms [35].

DOT Regimens for Tuberculosis is shown in Tables 2 and 3.

Table.2. 6 Month regimens (mgs / kg body wt daily).

Drug	Phase 1 (2 months).	Phase 2 (4 months)
Isoniazid	5	5
Rifampicin	10	10
Pyrazinamide	30	10
Streptomycin	15	
Ethambutol	25	

Table.3. 8 month regimen (mgs / kg body wt daily).

Drug	Phase 1 (2 months).	Phase 2 (4 months)
Isoniazid	5	5
Rifampicin	10	
Pyrazinamide	30	
Thiacetazone	2.5	
(together with Streptomycin	15	
Or Ethambutol	25 (15 mgs. in case of children)	

References

[1] Grange JM. Tuberculosis; Bacterial infections. In, *Topley and Wilson's Microbiology and Microbial Infections* 1998 ; 9th ed. Vol 3, 21: 391-417. Eds: William J Hausler Jr and Max Sussman . Arnold, London

[2] Stead WW, Bates JH. Evidence of a silent bacillemia in primary tuberculosis. *Ann Intern Med* 1971 ;74 :559

[3] Kochi, A. (1991). The global tuberculosis situation and the new control strategy of the World Health Organization. *Tubercle* 72, 1–6.

[4] Haas Francois, Sheila Sperber Haas. The origins of mycobacterium tuberculosis and the notion of its contagiuosness . in, *Tuberculosis.* 1996 ;1st ed. 1: pp 3-19. Eds .William N Rom, Stuart M Garay . Little Brown and Company London

[5] Bates H Joseph. The Tuberculin skin Test and Preventive Treatment for Tuberculosis. In, *Tuberculosis* Ist ed 1996 ; 865-871.eds. William N Rom , Stuart M Garay. Little Brown and company, London

[6] Centers for Disease Control. Screening for Tuberculosis and tuberculous infection with high risk populations and the use of preventive treatment for tuberculous infection in the US. Recommendations of the advisory committe for the elimination of tuberculosis MMWR 1990; 39: (No. RR-8): 1-12

[7] Satyanarayana BV . "Tuberculoderma" A brief review together with statistical analysis and observations. *Ind J Dermatol Venereol* 1963 Jan-March ; vol 29: No 1

[8] Lahiri KD. Etiology and pathology of skin tuberculosis in the tropics. *Int J Dermatol* 1956; 2: 3-7

[9] Sehgal VN, Srivastava G, Khuran VK , Sharma VK, Bhalla P, Beohar PC. An appraisal of epidemiologic , clinical, bacteriologic, histopathologic and immunologic parameters in cutaneous tuberculosis. *Int J Dermatol* 1987 ; 26 : 521

[10] Kumar B, Muralidhar S. Cutaneous tuberculosis – A twenty year prospective study. *Int J Tuberc Lung Dis* 1999 Jun ; 3 (6): 494-500

[11] Marmelzat WL. Laennec and the "prosector's wart". Arch Dermatol : 74 - 76

[12] Harahap Marwali . Tuberculosis of the skin. *Int J Dermatol* 1983, Nov ; Vol 22: No 9 pp542-545

[13] Good RC, Shinnick TM. Mycobacterium. In, *Topley And Wilson's Microbiology And Microbial Infections* 1998 ; 9th edition, volume 2 : 26 : 549-576 Editors. Albert Balows, Brian I Duerden. Published by Arnold, London

[14] Woods GL, Washington JA iii. Mycobacteria other than *Mycobacterium tuberculosis:* Review of microbiologic and clinical aspects. Rev Infect Dis 1987; 9:275-299

[15] Youmans GP. The morphology and metabolism of mycobacteria. In, Tuberculosis. 1979; pp8. W B Saunder's Company, Philadelphia

[16] Jenkins PA. Lipid analysis for the identification of mycobacteria : an appraisal. *Reviews of Infectious diseases* 1981; 3: 862-866

[17] Adler JJ, Rose DN. Transmission and Pathogenesis of tuberculosis. In Tuberculosis.1996. pp129-140 Eds: ROM and GARAY. Little Brown and Company. New York. USA

[18] Wolinsky E. Tuberculosis. In, *Textbook Of Pulmonary Diseases* 1994 (5th ed) ; pp521-573 Eds. GL Baum, E Wolinsky, Little Brown. Boston

[19] Robbins L. Infectious diseases. In, *Pathologic Basis Of Disease*. 1994; 5th ed . pp324-325. Eds. Stanley L Robbins, Ramzi S Cotran, Vinay Kumar . WB Saunders Co. Philadelphia

[20] Toossi Zahra, Jerrold Ellner. Host Response to Mycobacterium Tuberculosis. *Frontiers In Biosciences*.1998 July; 3: e133-140

[21] Hunter SW, Gaylord H, Brennan PJ. Structure and antigenicity of the phosphorylated lipopolysacharide antigens from the leprosy and tubercle bacilli. *J Biol Chem* 1986; 261 : 12345-12351

[22] Dahl KE, Shiratsuchi H, Hamilton BD, EllnerJJ, TossiZ. Selective induction of TGFb in human monocytes by LAM of M. tuberculosis. *Infect Immun.* 1996;64:399-405

[23] Wolff K, Tappeiner G. Mycobacterial diseases : tuberculosis and atypical mycobacterial infections. In, *Dermatology In General Medicine*, 1987 : 2152-2170. Eds. Fitzpatrick TB, Eisen AZ, Wolff K et al, New York: McGraw Hill

[24] Collins CH, Grange JM, Yates MD. *Organization And Practice In Tuberculosis Bacteriology* 1985; 1st Edn 1-2 Publishers- Butterworths

[25] Savin JA . Mycobacterial infections. In, *Textbook Of Dermatology*.1992 5th edition.; 1033. Eds. Champion RH, Burton JL, Ebling FJG. Blackwell Scientific Publications, London

[26] Smith DW, Weigeshaus EH, Navalkar R, Grover AA. Host-parasite relationships in experimental airborne tuberculosis. I preliminary studies in BCG vacinated and non-vaccinated animals. *J Bacteriol* 1966 ; 91:718-724

[27] Sehgal VN, Wagh SA. Cutaneous tuberculosis : current concepts. *Int J Dermatol* 1990 ; 29: 237-252

[28] Cruickshank Robert, Duguid JP, Marmion BP, Swain RHA. Mycobacterium Tuberculosis. In, *Medical Microbiology* 1973; 12th ed. vol 1(22) : 285-296 Churchill Livingstone. London.

[29] Rook GAW. The role of vitamin D in Tuberculosis . *Am Rev Resp Dis* 1988 ;10 : 231-49

[30] Kuhn Charles , Askin B Frederic. Lung and mediastinum .in, *Anderson's Pathology* 1985, 8th edition Vol 1; 22: pp 833-954. Editors John M Kissane and WAD Anderson. The CV Mosby company St Louis Missouri

[31] Rook GAW, Bloom BR. Mechanisms of pathogenesis of tuberculosis. In, *Tuberculosis* . 1994; 485. Eds Bloom BR. Pathogenesis, protection and control.. American Society for Microbiology Press Washington ,DC

[32] Dannenberg AM. Immune mechanisms in the pathogenesis of pulmonary tuberculosis. *Rev Infect Dis* 1989; 11: S 369

[33] *Lever's Histopathology of The Skin Eds*. David Elder, Rosalie Elenitsas, Christine Jaworsky, and Bernett Johnson. 1997 (8th ed) ; 21: p 468 Lippincott-Raven Philadelphia

[34] Sehgal VN, Gupta R, Bose M, Saha K. Immunohistopathological spectrum in cutaneous tuberculosis. *Clin Exptl Dermatol* 1993 ; 18: 309

[35] Kakakhel Khadim Ullah, Peter Fritsch. Cutaneous Tuberculosis. *Int J Dermatol* 1989, July- August; Vol 28: 355-362

[36] Beyt B Eugene, David W Ortbals, Daniel J, Santa Cruz, George S Kobayashi, Arthur Z Eisen, Gerald Medoff. Cutaneous Mycobacteriosis: An analysis of 34 cases with a New Classification of the Disease. *Medicine* 1980; vol 60:No 2 pp95-109

[37] Savin JA and Wilkinson DS. Mycobacterial infections including tuberculosis, in Text Book of Dermatology, 4th edition. Eds. Rook A, Wilkinson DS, Ebling FJD, Oxford *Blackwell* Scientific Publications, 1986:798-822

[38] Vero F. Primary inoculation tuberculosis of the skin with involvement of the regional lymph nodes. *Arch Dermatol Syphilol* 1941; 44 : 785

[39] Rubin EH. Hematogenous tuberculosis in the adult - Generalised hematogenous tuberculosis . *Am Rev Tuberc* 1937 ; 39 : 557

[40] Lantos Gabor, Benjamin K `, Monica Contreras. Tuberculous Ulcer of the skin. *J Am* Acad Dermatol 1988;19:1067-72

[41] Heilman KM, Muschenheim C. Primary cutaneous tuberculosis resulting from mouth to mouth respiration. *N Engl J Med* 1965 ; 273:1035

[42] Fisher JR. Miliary tuberculosis with unusual cutaneous manifestations. Jama 1977; 238:241-3

[43] Goette DK, Jacobson KW, Doty RD. Primary inoculation tuberculosis of the skin. *Arch Dermatol.* 1978;114:567–569

[44] Thompson BC. The pathogenesis of tuberculosis of peripheral lymph nodes. *Tubercle* 1940 ; 21: 217-35 and 260-68

[45] Miller FJW, Cashman JM. Origin of peripheral tuberculous lymphadenitis in childhood. *Lancet* 1958; 1: 286-89

[46] Findlay George Hudson. Bacterial Infections. In, *The Dermatology Of Bacterial Infections.* 1987 1st ed ; pp 71 - 83 Blackwell scientific publications , London

[47] Visser VJ, Heyl T. Skin tuberculosis as seen at GaRankuwa hospital. *Clin Expt Dermatol* 1993 ;18 : 507-515

[48] Golden Richard L. Sir William Osler and the anatomical tubercle. *J Am Acad Dermatol* 1987; vol 16: no 5: part 1 1071-74

[49] Wong KD, Lee KP, Chiu SF. Tuberculosis of the skin in Hong Kong (A review of 160 cases). *Br J Dermatol* 1968; 80: 424 –429

[50] Singh Gurmohan. Lupus Vulgaris in India . *Ind J Dermatol And Venereol* 1974 ; vol 40:No 6, 257-260

[51] Mitchell PC. Tuberculosis verrucosa cutis among Chinese in Hong Kong. *Br J Dermatol* 1954; 66: 444

[52] Michelson E Henry. Criteria for the diagnosis of certain tuberculodermas. *The J Am Med Ass* 1948 Nov; Vol 138: No(10) 721-25

[53] Mehregan Amir H . Predominantly Mononuclear granulomas. *In Pinkus' Guide To Dermatohistopathology.* 1986 4th ed ; 21: pp254-255 Appleton-Century-Crofts/Norwalk,Connecticut

[54] Ulcerative Lupus Vulgaris-Face -- an uncommon presentation in India. *Indian J Tuberc.* 2007; 54(1):52-4.

[55] Psoriasiform lupus vulgaris . L Padmavathy, L Lakshmana Rao, N.Ethirajan, M.Dhanalakshmi- *Ind J Tuberculosis* 2008; 55: 97-99

[56] Rubin EH. Hematogenous tuberculosis in the adult - Generalised hematogenous tuberculosis . *Am Rev Tuberc* 1937 ; 39 : 557

[57] Callahan F Elizabeth, Anita L Licata, Jennifer F Madison. Cutaneous *Myc obacterium kansasi* infection associated with a papulonecrotic tuberculid reaction. *J Am Acad Dermatol* 1997; 36:497-9

[58] Wilson–Jones E, Winkelman RK. Papulonecrotic tuberculid: A neglected disease in western countries. *J Am Acad Dermatol* 1986;14:815-826

[59] Sloan(1990)

[60] Degitz K, Steidl M, Thomas P, Plewig G, Volkenandt M. Aetiology of tuberculids. *The Lancet* 1993 Jan 23; vol 341

[61] Singh Gurmohan, Sanjay Singh, Vineet Kaur. in, *Iadvl Text Book And Atlas Of Dermatology* 1994 ;Vol 1, No 10: 164-172 , eds. RG Valia and AR Valia. Bhalani Publishing house Bombay.

[62] Rademaker M, Lowe DG, Munro DD. Erythema Induratum (Bazin's Disease). *J Am Acad Dermatol* 1989; 21 : 740-745

[63] Yen Angela, Paul Fearneyhough, Peter Rady, Stephen Tyring , Dayna diven. Erythema induratum of Bazin as a tuberculid: Confirmation of *Mycobacterium tuberculosis* DNA Polymerase Chain Reaction analysis. *J Am Acad Dermatol* 1997; 36 : 99-101

[64] Ackerman B. *Histologic diagnosis of inflammatory skin diseases*, 1978; Lea and Febriger. Philadelphia

[65] Moschella SL. Benign reticuloendothelial diseases. In, *Dermatology* 1985; Vol 1 : 751 . eds. Moschella SL, Pillsbury DM, Hurley HJ. WB Saunder's companyy, Philadelphia-London

[66] Yanez MA, Coppola MP, Russo DA. Determination of mycobacterial antigens in sputum by Enzyme Immuno Assay. *J Clin Microbiol* 1986; 23 : 822-825

[67] Sehgal VN, Ahuja P, Sharma VK. Cell - mediated immunity in cutaneous tuberculosis. *Br J Dermatol* 1988 ; 118 : 730

[68] Centers for Diseases Control. Anergy skin testing and preventive therapy for HIV infected persons-*Revised Recommendations* 1997 Sept 5; 46(RR15):1-10

[69] Rook GAW. The role of vitamin D in Tuberculosis . *Am Rev Resp Dis* 1988 ;10 : 231-49

[70] Strauss E, Wu N. Radioimmuno assay of tuberculoprotein derived from *Mycobacterium tuberculosis. Proc Natl Acad Sci Usa* 1980; 77: 4301-4304

[71] Strauss E, Wu N , Quraishi MAH, Levine S. Clinical applications of the radioimmunoassay of secretory tuberculoprotein. *Proc Natl Acad Sci Usa* 1981; 78: 3214-3217

[72] Daniel TM. Rapid diagnosis of tuberculosis : Laboratory techniques applicable in developing countries. *Rev Infect Dis* 1989 ;11(Suppl 2):5471-5478

[73] Drake TA, Hindler JA, Berlin OGW, Bruckner DA. Rapid identification of *Mycobacterium avium* complex in culture using DNA probes. *J Clin Microbiol* 1987; 25: 1442-1445

[74] Goto M , Oka S, Okuzumi K, et al. Evaluation of Acridinium –ester –labelled DNA probes for identification of *Mycobacterium tuberculosis* and *Mycobacterium avium – Mycobacterium intracellulare complex* in culture. *J Clin Microbiol* 1991; 29: 2473-2476

[75] Portillo PD, Murillo LA, Patarroyo ME. Amplification of species-specific DNA fragment of *Mycobacterium tuberculosis* and its possible use in diagnosis . *J Clin Microbiol* 1991; 29: 2163-2168

[76] Kocakoz T, Engin Yilmazz, Seref Ozkara, Sesin Kocakoz, Murat Hayran, Meena Sachedeva, & Henry F Chambers. Detection of *Mycobacterium tuberculosis* in sputum samples by Polymerase Chain Reaction using a simplified procedure. *J Clin Microbiol* 1993 June; 31: 1435-1438

[77] Polymerase Chain reaction (PCR) as a diagnostic tool in cutaneous tuberculosis *–Ijdvl.* 2003; 69 (3): 214-216

[78] Cersello BF. New approach to treatment of pulmonary and extra pulmonary tuberculosis. *Int J Dermatol* 1987; 26: 185-189

[79] Centers for Disease Control. Screening for tuberculosis and tuberculous infection with high risk populations and the use of preventive treatment for tuberculous infection in the US. Recommendations of the advisory committee for the elimination of tuberculosis *Mmwr.* 1990;39☹n0.RR-8):1-12

[80] Iseman MD, Sharbaro JA. National ACCP conference on tuberculosis . *Chest* 1985 ; 87 : 115S - 149S

Chapter XIII

Suppurative Lesions Complicating Chronic Anal Fissures

PJ Gupta

Gupta Nursing Home, Laxminagar, Nagpur, India

Abstract

Suppurative pathologies associated with chronic anal fissures are common but are not well documented. Fissure abscess, post fissure fistula, and post fissure antibioma are but a few of them. These pathologies increase the complications and morbidity of the primary lesion and need a comprehensive approach. From the hospital case record of 532 patients treated for chronic anal fissures, 88 (16.5%) were found to have one of these pathologies. This retrospective study describes such pathologies in terms of demographics, clinical presentation, pathological features, operative technique and the outcome. 95% of the patients presented with pain and discharge per anus. Following the surgical procedure, 90% of them could resume their duties within a week. Wound healing took a period between 2 weeks to 2 months. At the last follow up at 18 months, three patients had a recurrence (3.4%). Suppuration in chronic anal fissure seems to be more frequent than described. While dealing with the anal fissure, it is desirable to look for these associated pathologies as well to avoid complications and morbidity of the primary disease.

Keywords: Anal fissure. Fissure abscess. Post fissure fistula. Suppuration.

Introduction

Fissure in ano is a very common disease of the anal canal. In most cases, it is more annoying than dangerous. Diagnosis is easy and most patients have a typical history of pain and anal bleeding. Local examination is sufficient to clinch the diagnosis. The treatment is based on reducing the spasm of the internal anal sphincter, employing various medical therapies or surgical techniques [1].

Problem often arises when the fissure gets complicated due to invasion by suppurative pathogens. These organisms lead to a purulent infection in and around the anal fissure causing paraproctitis, abscess or anal fistula [2].

The present retrospective study is a brief description of some of these pathologies in respect to their clinical presentation, operative procedure performed and the outcome of the treatment.

The aim of this study was to assess the incidence of suppuration in chronic anal fissures and to evaluate the outcome of the surgical procedures performed in such pathologies.

Although, these pathologies do not manifest with a typical natural history and presentation, but a clinical distinction between them is necessary because the treatment plan differs in each of these pathologies. Few of the more common of these are discussed below.

Fissure abscess- It is a subcutaneous abscess lying in immediate periphery of an anal fissure [3]. It develops due to gathering of granulating tissues around edges of the fissure. Undermining between this and the internal sphincter a small abscess is formed, which is just superficial to the internal sphincter. The abscess is unable to drain due to anal sphincter spasm. At times, an external skin tag may itself become undermined distally, forming a bridged fissure draining pus underneath (superficial fistula)[4].

Nevertheless, a small abscess in the intersphincteric space at the middle of the anal canal causes pain very similar to that of fissure and the diagnosis may be delayed because few physical signs are present [5]. However, a tender nodule can be discovered on local examination. This is an abscess, which remains localized to the primary site in the anal canal and does not spread. (Figure 1)

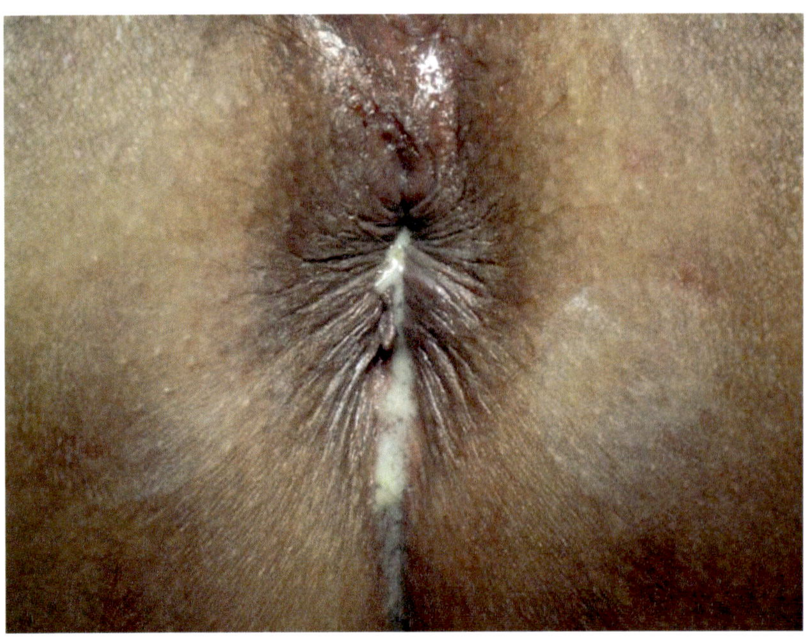

Figure1- A fissure abscess.

At times, it is difficult to differentiate the pain of an abscess from that of anal fissure. As against a throbbing pain caused by an abscess, the pain in fissure is not a continuous one and is mostly associated with defecation. Inguinal adenopathy is seen with the abscess and not with fissure alone.

Post fissure anal fistula- A superficial fistula occurs in association with a chronic anal fissure and runs subcutaneously or under a sentinel tag if present. Unlike in the usual anal fistula, pain is a leading symptom. The fistula is very close to the anal orifice, mostly placed posteriorly and the external opening may be hidden under the sentinel pile. In addition, there may be an inflammatory swelling behind the fissure secondary to an intersphincteric or perianal abscess. A probe can be passed through the external opening, which emerges out through the fissure. [6] (Figure 2)

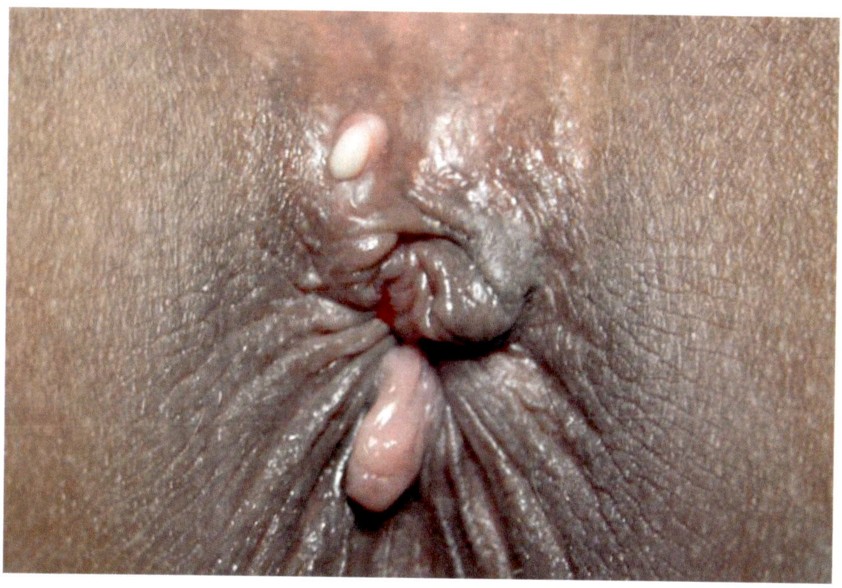

Figure 2. Post fissure fistula.

Post-Fissure Antibioma

The entity has a characteristic history. It occurs due to inadequate or delayed drainage of the anal abscess, which assumes chronicity. This abscess is not incised in time and is treated only with antibiotics. This causes the abscess to be walled off with fibrotic tissue forming an'*antibioma'* (antibiotic granuloma, organized abscess, sterile abscess) which may mimic a neoplastic mass. The lump is usually tender, but not always so. Patient may have tender lymph nodes in the inguinal region. (Figure 3)

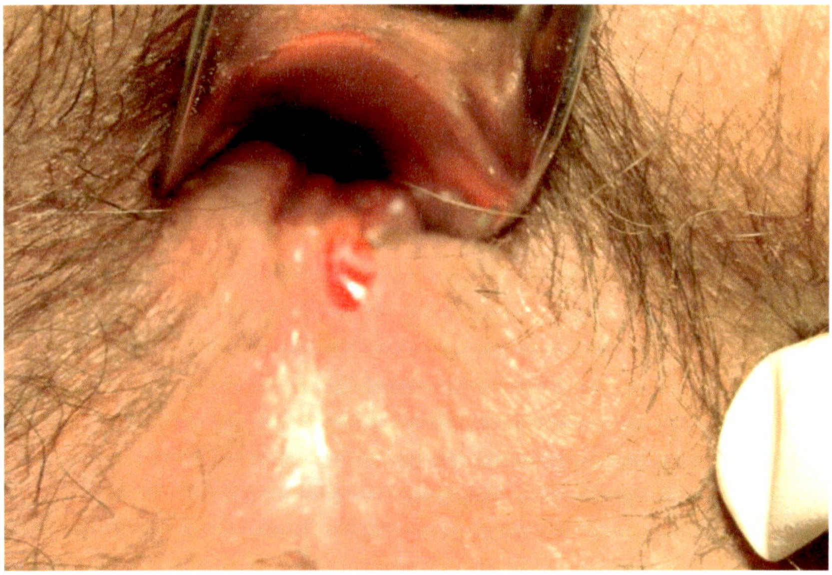

Figure 3. Post fissure antibioma.

Pyogenic Granuloma

Pyogenic granuloma is a common, acquired, benign vascular lesion of skin and mucous membranes, which may occasionally present intravascularly or subcutaneously. Proposed agents include trauma, infection, and preceding dermatoses. In the anal site it appears as a sessile or peduncolated, red-wine, soft little tumor of the size of a millet or barley grain (inflammatory hyperplasia). (Figure 4)

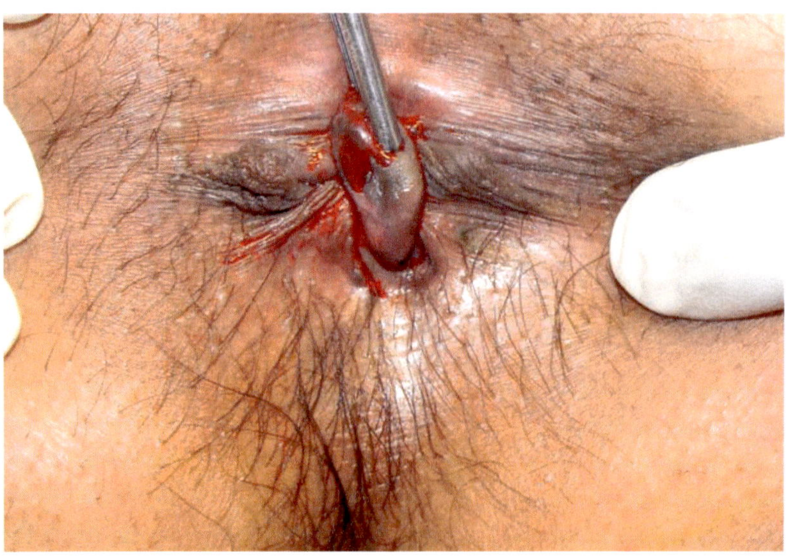

Figure 4- Post fissure granuloma.

The condition may persist for years together with remission and relapses. The symptomatic presentation is by intermittent discharge per anus or a sense of heaviness in the anal canal. Occasionally, it may burst open internally with a small opening, which causes pruritus and perianal soiling. The diagnosis can be made by eliminating the other causes of a tender, firm to hard lump and by obtaining a negative culture report of the discharge.

Materials and Methods

A data was collected from the medical records at Gupta Nursing Home, Nagpur, India for a period of 8 years from July 1998 to June 2006. Patients with chronic anal fissures were sorted out. The criteria for diagnosis of chronic anal fissure were-

1. Unresponsiveness of anal fissure to conservative treatment.
2. Presence of an external skin tag.
3. Induration at the edges of fissure.
4. Visible fibers of the internal sphincter at the floor of the fissure.
5. Fissure base showing features of infection.
6. Pus discharge from the fissure.

Inclusion Criteria

Patients of chronic anal fissure having history of pus discharge, presence of a subcutaneous fistula in the close vicinity and those having a palpable, tender lump at the base of the fissure were selected for this study irrespective of the duration of disease.

Exclusion Criteria

Patients having associated hemorrhoids, anal fistulae at other places than near the fissure and those who were on steroids or immuno-suppressant drugs were not included. Similarly, patients who did not report during the follow-up schedule were kept out of the study.

Preoperative Investigations

All the patients were screened for HIV, apart from the routine hematological tests like leukocyte count and ESR.

None of the patient was subjected to endoanal ultrasonography, fistulography or MRI, as none was felt necessary. Clinical examination was found sufficient to make the diagnosis.

The factors analyzed were 1) demographics, 2) presenting symptoms, 3) operative procedure, 4) postoperative results and 5) follow-up findings.

Operative Treatment

An informed consent was obtained from all the patients. This study was approved by the local ethical committee and was performed according to the declaration of Helsinki.

30 cc of Lactulose solution was administered orally on the night before the procedure. All the procedures were carried out under a short general anesthesia

A radiofrequency surgical procedure was performed to tackle these associated pathologies.

Radiofrequency- Radio frequency surgery involves cutting or coagulation of tissues by using a high frequency alternate current.

A radiofrequency generator Ellman dual frequency 4 MHz (Ellman International, Oceanside, N.Y. USA) was used. This instrument produces an electromagnetic wave of a very high frequency that reaches 4 megahertz. The unit is supplied with a handle to which different inter changeable electrodes could be attached to suit the requirement. In our procedure, a ball electrode for coagulation, a round loop electrode to shave off the offending tissues and a fine needle electrode to incise the skin were used.

Fissure abscess- The abscess cavity was incised with the needle electrode of the radiofrequency device and the pus evacuated. The edges of the incision were trimmed with a loop electrode making it into a pear shaped wound tapering towards the anal canal. This facilitated free drainage and avoided possibility of developing a fistula later. After irrigation of the cavity with antiseptic, it was lightly packed with gauze.

Post fissure Fistula- A probe was passed from the external opening to bring it out from the internal one. The skin over the probe was coagulated with the ball electrode. This reduced bleeding during incision of the tract. With a needle electrode, the tract was slit opened. The edges of the wound were trimmed to give it a pear shape tapering towards the anus.

Post fissure Antibioma- The skin over the lump was incised with the needle electrode. Then with the help of the loop electrode, the entire indurated mass and hard tissue from the lump was shaved off leaving a red raw area behind.

Results

The present study describes 88 cases of suppurative pathologies found amongst 532 cases of chronic anal fissure (16.5%) treated during 8 year's period. In 349 (66%) patients, the fissure was in the posterior midline, while in 117(22%) patients it was found in the anterior midline position. 66(12%) patients had fissures on both ends of the midline. Out of the 88 patients who had associated suppurative pathologies, 53 (60%) were males. The mean age of the patients was 37 (range 20- 44). The mean duration of disease was 23 months. The incidence of abscess was highest (42%) while that of post fissure antibioma was least (19%). The incidence of pathologies was found to be higher in the posterior midline than those found in the anterior midline position (70:30). Four of these 88 patients were suffering from diabetes and were under treatment. No other co-morbid conditions like jaundice, uremia, or systemic infection was found. All the patients treated were found to be negative for HIV virus.

Table 1. Patient Demographic (n=88).

Male	53(60.2%)	
Female	35(39.8 %)	
Mean duration of disease (months) (range)	23 months (5-45)	
Mean age of the patients (years) (range)	37 (20-44yrs)	
Post fissure abscess	37 (42.1%)	Posterior 26 (70%) Anterior 11 (30%)
Post fissure fistula	34 (38.6%)	Posterior 23 (68%) Anterior 11 (32%)
Post fissure antibioma	17 (19.3%)	Posterior 12 (71%) Anterior 5 (29%)

All the patients received medical treatment in the past. The prescribed medicines mostly contained antibiotics, analgesics, local applications of antiseptics and anesthetic ointments and laxatives. Two patients having fistula gave history of being operated in the past by posterior sphincterotomy.

The clinical presentation was of varied type. (Table 2)

Table 2. Clinical presentation of patients with suppurative pathologies (n= 88).

Pain	85 (96.6%)
Discharge	59 (67%)
Pruritus	53 (60%)
Sentinel tag	34 (38.6%)
Bleeding	18 (20.4%)
Sense of incomplete evacuation	17 (19.3%)
Inguinal lymphadenopathy	7 (7.9%)

Pain- All but three of the 88 patients complained of pain, which was predominantly post defecation and lasting for about 2 hrs. Those having abscess had a continuous, throbbing type of pain, which compelled them to seek surgeon's advice at an early date. The remaining 3 patients had no pain but had complaint of discharge per anus.

Discharge- Fifty-nine patients complained of discharge from the anus. In majority of cases, it was scanty in amount, causing soiling of the underclothes, but in 13 patients, it was profuse and offensive in odor.

Pruritus- Fifty-three patients complained of itching in and around the anus. In 34 of them, the pruritus was continuous, while it was predominantly post defecation in the remaining 19 patients.

Sentinel pile- Thirty-four patients had an external pile. Twenty- one of these was edematous while in 13 it was in a shrunken state. 16 had a fistulous opening beneath them.

Bleeding- The incidence of bleeding in the studied patients was less as compared to other symptoms. Only 18 of them had post defecation bleeding.

The other complaints noticed were- sense of incomplete evacuation and inguinal lymphadinopathy.

Follow-up- (Table 3)

Table 3. Post procedure follow-up findings.

Follow-up after 2 weeks	
Pain	32
Bleeding	3
Discharge	14
Time to resume work	4 days (range 2-10 days)
Follow-up after 4 weeks	
Anal spasm	None
Presence of wound	8
Follow-up after 8 weeks	
Lymphadinopathy	None
Wound	None
Follow-up after 18 months.	
Recurrence of fissure	2
Recurrence of pus discharge	1

At a first follow up after 2 weeks, 32 patients still had a burning pain, which was beginning at defecation and lasting for a mean of 12 minutes. The mean analgesic dose requirement for each patient was 26 (range 20- 38).

Three patients complained of bleeding from the wound. On inspection, it was found that the wounds were showing hypergranulation. The granulation was scrapped and they were advised not to apply any ointment over the wound. They were asked to discontinue sitz bath also. This relieved the bleeding and complete healing was achieved.

Fourteen patients still had a discharge from the wounds. In 9 of them, it was scanty and odorless, but the other 5 had a profuse and foul smelling discharge. The discharge was sent for culture and sensitivity, and appropriate antibiotics were prescribed. The discharge ceased thereafter.

Twelve patients complained of incontinence for flatus, but none of them had any incontinence for feces.

The mean period off work was 4 days (range 2- 10 days). Patients treated for abscess were able to resume duties between 2 and 5 days. However, those having fistula or antibioma took a period of 4 to 10 days to return to their routine.

At 4-week follow-up, per rectal digital examination and anoscopy was performed. None of the patients was found to have any sphincter spasm. The wounds of patients with abscess and fistula were healed, but 8 patients who were operated for antibioma, the wounds were yet to heal. One patient operated for fistula had a premature skin closure, which was slit opened. It healed uneventfully thereafter. 2 patients still had incontinence for flatus.

At 8 weeks, the wounds in all the patients were healed. Those having enlarged lymph nodes in the inguinal region showed complete regression of the same. Two patients, who had incontinence for flatus, got relieved of the embarrassing complaint.

At the follow-up after 18 months of the procedure, 2 patients had recurrence of fissure. They were prescribed nitroglycerine ointment. One patient, who was operated for antibioma, had recurrence of pus discharge. He refused to undergo further treatment. (Table 4)

Table 4. Complication rate.

Complication	No of patients (incidence rate)
Incontinence to flatus	12 (13.6%)
Hypergranulation of wounds	3 (3.4%)
Premature skin closure of fistula wound	1 (2.9%)
Re-infection in antibioma	1 (5.8%)
Recurrence of fissure	2 (2.2)

Discussion

Suppurative lesions are not uncommon to be found with chronic anal fissure. The theory of a crypto glandular infection as the cause of perianal suppuration seems to be realistic [7]. Most of the purulent pathologies are due to diseases of the anal glands, which become chronically infected. Some are probably the results of infection in the lymphoid tissues found around the anal glands [8]. The chronic anal fissure likewise represents a pathogenetic factor in the genesis of sepsis, especially in the posterior part of the anal canal. In this region one can find supra and trans- sphincteric tracts with abscesses in the fossa ischiorectalis [9].

Anal cryptitis is the first member of a chain of inflammatory sequel. It is frequently overlooked, yet in the early stages it could easily be managed by suitable conservative measures [10]. Nevertheless, when organisms creep in, the infection extends in the depth and circumference. This may cause frank suppuration leading to an abscess formation, or may remain in dormancy as an antibioma or fistula with intermittent bouts of flare-ups.

Majority of them presents with pain and discharge. Study by Sainio accounted 3.3% of anal fistula originating in the anal fissure [11].

In India, the incidences of these pathologies seem to be relatively more common as patients with symptoms referable to the anorectum do not seek medical attention early [12]. Those seeking medical advice are initially treated by their family physicians. These include Allopaths, Homoeopaths and Ayurvedic doctors. On being implored, it was found that the patients under our study were prescribed antibiotics and anti-inflammatory medicines for long durations. This probably had masked the acute symptoms and led the suppurative process to lie in a state of dormancy. The post fissure abscess treated with antibiotics might have ' sterilized' and walled off to persist as an antibioma, or had burst opened to give rise to a fistula.

These entities cause a significant nuisance, with frequent episodes of suppuration, pruritus and foreign body sensation in the anus. It is important to remove all the tissues at the primary site so that infected glandular lymphoid tissue is completely extirpated. Pruritus and discharge occurred significantly more often in patients with a longer duration of symptoms and those with pruritus and drainage were mostly having a fistula. Patients with chronic anal pruritus or an anal abscess are required to be carefully evaluated for an anal fistula, since anorectal problems may recur if a fistula remains untreated. [13]

No attempt was made for primary closure of the wounds, to avoid risks like persistence of dead space or wound dehiscence. The wounds were allowed to heal by second intention. [14] Timely diagnosis of combined pathology helps in preventing the development of possible complications and in choosing the most helpful surgical tactics in every specific case [15]. Reports have favored excision of the anal fissure in case of fissures with intersphincteric fistula or abscess [16].

Though our study showed that the incidence of suppurative pathologies associated with chronic anal fissure was 16.5%, in actuality, it was a little more i.e., 18.5%, but as 2% of the patients could not be traced during the follow-ups, we have not included them in this study.

Though the incidence of occurrence of anal fissure is equal in both males and females, in our study however, the number of male patients was more than the females. The probable explanation to this discrepancy is the reluctance of the females of India to get them examined and treated for these diseases.

The present trend of treatment for anal fissure is inclined towards pharmacological manipulation of the internal sphincter using various drugs or by applying nitroglycerine ointment or injecting botulinum toxin. However, these would not be effective in anal fissures complicated by an abscess, fistula or antibioma. Presumably, such non- operative approaches for chronic anal fissure avoids anesthesia and surgical intervention, but the associated lesions cannot be eliminated by mere conservation. Surgical management is more effective in respect to the time factor [17] where a timely decision to intervene will considerably improve the overall outcome [18].

Though these procedures can be performed with the conventional techniques, we have opted for radiofrequency surgery, as this technique simultaneously achieves cutting and coagulation. This attribute of the tool minimizes bleeding and allows an effortless curettage of infected tissues. [19] Complete extirpation of the offending tissue helps in faster and smoother recovery with reduced chances of recurrence. [20]

As reported by others, we have not encountered a single case developing a keyhole deformity, which is feared after removal of the fissure while dealing with the suppurative pathologies [21]. None of the patients operated for post fissure abscess developed any fistula in the subsequent follow up in our study.

Patients who were operated for fistula or antibioma took a little more time to resume routine than those operated for abscess. This probably was due to prompt relief of pain after drainage of pus, while the wounds of fistula and antibioma were relatively more painful after the procedure than before.

These perianal infections could at times, be an effect of the treatment of the fissure it self. Surgical procedures like sphincterotomy or injection of botulinum toxin are fraught with complications like ano rectal sepsis, causing abscess and fistula. [22-23] Two of the patients in this study gave history of being previously operated by posterior sphincterotomy and subsequently developed a fistula.

A symptomatic HIV infection is an important determinant of progress after surgery. [24] There is a significant prevalence of anorectal sepsis and secondary anal fissurations in homosexual men. The causes of the sepsis in such situation are multiple. The most frequent is infectious, and essentially, a sexually transmitted disease [25]. A report describes of a homosexual male patient who presented with perianal abscess that was caused by infection with Neisseria gonorrhoeae. [26]

Uncommonly, tumors of the perianal region and anal canal can also mimic like an abscess or antibioma. They can present in a variety of ways, most frequently as a painful lump close to the anal margin. Recurrent suppuration and discharge through an external opening is another presentation. They could be malignant as in case of a primary perianal mucinous adenocarcinoma;or benign like a leiomyoma or an aggressive angiomyxoma. [27] We however, did not come across such tumors in our study.

Patients with immuno-compromised status are more prone for ano rectal sepsis. A careful search to find out such condition in patients showing slow wound healing or recurrent suppuration is mandatory. Existence of such entity can lead to recurrence or chronic problem wounds [28].

Though a good digital examination is usually sufficient for the diagnosis and the treatment planning of anal fistulae, cross-sectional imaging techniques, however, can accurately identify deep abscesses and characterize existence of anal fistulae. Magnetic resonance (MR) imaging has been shown to demonstrate accurately the anatomy of the perianal region as well as the location of deep abscesses, the state of the ano-rectal wall and the perirectal spaces, and the damages of the anal sphincter [29,30].

A chronic anal fissure is often associated with hyperhidrosis of the anal fold and perianal skin. This occasionally can lead to Hidradenitis Suppurativa (HS), an uncommon disorder frequently involving the perianal region. This represents a chronic, recurrent, deep-seated folliculitis resulting in abscesses followed by the formation of sinus tracts and scarring [31]. The disease at times presents with multiple site involvement like the axilla, nape of the neck and perianal region. The pathology can be confirmed by histological examination, which shows epidermis-lined sinuses surrounded by dense plasma cell infiltration.

As in all of the procedures described above, the fibers of internal sphincter needed to be severed, no additional sphincterotomy or anal stretch was found necessary to relieve the anal spasm.

The present study demonstrates that suppuration is common with chronic anal fissures, which can present as an abscess, fistula or antibioma. A careful search to rule out such association can avert more complex situations.

Conclusion

Infective pathologies associated with chronic anal fissure need a more aggressive approach. Surgical approach with radiofrequency was found to be effective in dealing with the types of pathologies discussed in this study.

References

[1] Dziki A, Trzcinski R, Langner E, Wronski W. New approaches to the treatment of anal fissure. *Acta Chir Iugosl.* 2002; 49: 73-75.
[2] Nazarov LU, Orgusian RV. Surgical procedure in combined proctologic diseases. Vestn Khir Im I I Grek. 1978; 121: 84-87.
[3] Lock MR. (1981) *Fissure* .In: Thomson J.P.S, Nicholls RJ, Williams C.B (edits), Colorectal diseases, William Heinemann Medical Book Limited, London, pp 345-346.
[4] Williams NS (1995) *The anus and anal canal.* In: Mann CV, Russell RCG, Williams NS (edits) Bailey & Love's short practice of surgery.22nd edition. Chapman & Hall, London, pp 879.
[5] Park AG, Thomson JP. Intersphincteric abscess. *Br Med J.* 1973; 2: 537-539.
[6] Goligher J. (1992) *Anal Fissure*. In: Goligher J, Duthie H, Nixon H (edts) Bailliere Tindall, London, pp153.
[7] Girona J, Denkers D. Fistula, fissure, abscess. Chirurg. 1996; 67: 222-228.
[8] Parks AG Thomson JPS. (1981) *Abscess and Fistula*. In: Thomson J.P.S, Nicholls RJ, Williams C.B (edits), Colorectal disease. William Heinemann Medical Book Limited, London: pp 321-328.
[9] Jostarndt L, Nitsche D, Thiede A, Schroder D. *Pathogenesis and morphology of anal fistulas*. Fortschr Med. 1984;102: 615-618.
[10] Hein KE. *Practical proctology*. MMW Munch Med Wochenschr. 1975;117: 1705-1708.
[11] Sainio P. Fistula-in-ano in a defined population. Incidence and epidemiological aspects. *Ann Chir Gynaecol.* 2002; 1984;73: 219-224.
[12] Gopal DV. Diseases of the rectum and anus: a clinical approach to common disorders. *Clin Cornerstone*. 1987; 4: 34-48.
[13] Petros JG, Rimm EB, Robillard RJ. Clinical presentation of chronic anal fissures. *Am Surg.* 1993; 59: 666-668.
[14] Bock JU, Jongen J. Proctologic surgery in ambulatory care. *Langenbecks Arch Chir* Suppl Kongressbd. 1991; 1:386-388.
[15] Nazarov LU, *Orgusian RV*. Surgical procedure in combined proctologic diseases Vestn Khir Im I I Grek. 1978; 121: 84-87.
[16] Hager T. Anal fissure. *Ther Umsch.* 1997; 54: 190-192.
[17] Oh JT, Han A, Han SJ, Choi SH, Hwang EH. Fistula-in-ano in infants: is nonoperative management effective? *J Pediatr Surg* . 2001; 36: 1367-1369.
[18] Gilliland R, Wexner SD. Complicated anorectal sepsis. *Surg Clin North Am*. 1997; 77: 115-153.

[19] Gupta PJ. Sphincterotomy with radio frequency surgery: a new treatment technique of fissure in ano and associated pathologies. *Rom J Gastroenterol.* 2003; 12: 37-40.

[20] Nicholls J. Fissure in ano and anorectal sepsis. *Verh Dtsch Ges Inn Med.* 1988; 94:225-229.

[21] Oueidat D. A comparative study in anal fissure treatment. *J Med Liban.* 1999; 47: 164-168.

[22] Lewis TH, Corman ML, Prager ED, Robertson WG. Long-term results of open and closed sphincterotomy for anal fissure. *Dis Colon Rectum.* 1988; 31: 368-371.

[23] Carditello A, Meduri F, Cardillo P, Mule V, La Rocca T, Caminiti F. Proctologic day-surgery. Results of 2000 surgical interventions. *Chir Ital.* 2001; 53: 219-224.

[24] Carr ND, Mercey D, Slack WW. Non-condylomatous, perianal disease in homosexual men. *Br J Surg.* 1989; 76: 1064-1066.

[25] Fellous K. Anal fissures and fissurations. Rev Prat. 2001; 51: 32-35.

[26] El-Dhuwaib Y, Ammori BJ. Perianal abscess due to Neisseria gonorrhoeae: an unusual case in the post-antibiotic era. *Eur J Clin Microbiol Infect Dis.* 2003; 22: 422-423.

[27] Bracey EE, Mathur P, Dooldeniya M, Joshi A, Dawson PM. Unusual perianal tumours masquerading as abscesses. *Int J Clin Pract.* 2003; 57: 343-346.

[28] Munoz-Villasmil J, Sands L, Hellinger M. Management of perianal sepsis in immunosuppressed patients. *Am Surg.* 2001; 67: 484-486.

[29] Morris J, Spencer JA, Ambrose NS. MR imaging classification of perianal fistulas and its implications for patient management. *Radiographics.* 2000; 20: 623-635.

[30] Cuenod CA, de Parades V, Siauve N, Marteau P, Grataloup C, Hernigou A, Berger A, Cugnenc PH, Frija G. MR imaging of ano-perineal sepsis. J Radiol. 2003; 84: 516-528.

[31] Endo Y, Tamura A, Ishikawa O, Miyachi Y. Perianal hidradenitis suppurativa: early surgical treatment gives good results in chronic or recurrent cases. *Br J Dermatol.* 1998; 139: 906-910.

Chapter XIV

Bird Flu in India

Introduction to Bird Flu [1 - 30]

Bird flu or atypical avian influenza is kind of influenza. The bird flu virus can cause the respiratory tract infection owing to the nature of general influenza. Basically, influenza virus can be classified into 3 groups: A, B and C. The classification relies mainly on the difference of nucleoprotein and matrix antigens [1 – 2]. In addition, influenza can also be divided into subtypes depending on hosts (Table 1). Influenza viruses have their spherical shape with average size about 1000 A in diameter and have an as yet undefined central structure containing the eight negative-sense RNA particles of the genome in association with the transcriptase required for mRNA synthesis, an abundant nucleoprotein, and a similarly abundant matrix protein [3]. This core is surrounded by a membrane got from the cell surface in a budding process by which newly formed viruses are secreted out from the infected cell [3]. During infection cell membranes are affected by the incorporation of newly synthesized virus membrane proteins [3]. As a result, the released viruses contain exclusively two different kinds of virus-specified glycoprotein, hemagglutinin and neuraminidase, and a proton channel protein, M2 [3]. As previously mentioned, the influenza viruses have segmented, negative stranded RNA genomes (vRNA) and are also enveloped [4]. The viruses can be derived from the plasma membrane of many cells especially for the apical plasma membrane of polarized epithelial cells [4]. Complete virus particles are not found inside infected cells [4]. Virus particles is composed of three major subviral components, namely the viral envelope, matrix protein (M1), and core (viral ribonucleocapsid [vRNP]) [4]. Several kinds of interactions that lead to virus assembly are described, including interactions between matrix proteins and membranes, interactions between matrix proteins and glycoproteins, interactions between matrix proteins and nucleocapsids, as well as interactions that lead to matrix protein self-assembly [5]. For viral morphogenesis to occur, all three viral components, namely the viral envelope, M1, and the vRNP have to be led to the assembly site at previously mentioned cells [4]. Finally, buds need to be created at the assembly site and virus particles released with the closure of buds [4]. These are important basic knowledge in virology of influenza virus.

Influenza group A is widely noted in medicine. Subtype classification of influenza group A virus can be set based on different of two main surface antigens, hemagglutin in (H) and neuraminidase (N). There are at least 16 H and 9 N forms. Of several kinds of influenza viruses, H5N1 is the specific cause of present epidemics in several region of the world. H5N1 turns to be the new focus at present. Hundreds of human infected cases were documented in medical literature. Pandemic of this new emerging virus infection is expected. H5N1 infection turns to be a new emerging infectious disease on medical surveillance. Similar to other infectious disorders in medicine, two main factors contributing to the emerging of bird flu are inherited and non-inherited factors. Basically, the inherited factor has been extensively looked for its role in response to many illnesses, especially for response to contagious illnesses. The effect of host genetic on the susceptibility to influenza virus has been studied for many years. Until present, it can be shown that the studies on host genetic susceptibility for bird flu are very limited therefore additional researches to discover new knowledge on this area are suggested. Besides the host susceptibility, the susceptibility of pathogen to anti-pathogenic agent is also broadly mentioned. Drug resistant influenza virus is reported and it is accepted that the H5N1 strains are highly resistant to amantadine and rimantadine but are susceptible to neuraminidase inhibitors, which can be used for treatment and prophylaxis. Genetic mutation and recombination are believed to be the most important factor leading to the emerging and possible pandemic of bird flu in human. It is noted that cross-species transmission events can result in a greater likelihood of a pandemic strain evolving than those caused by low-level transmission between humans [6].

Focusing on non-inherited factors, poverty should be mentioned. It is accepted that low income is a main barrier to good health service [7]. According to the outbreak of 1918-1919 influenza in the British Caribbean, the heaviest mortality rates were among the poor infected people [8]. The association between poverty and bird flu infection in humans is confirmed [9 - 11]. Therefore, the development based on the economic growth, to conquer the poverty in the tropical countries is required and become the politic strategies for all developing countries. As it is previously mentioned, poor hygiene can be the outcome of the poverty. It was found that predisposing factors of the village that might have influenced the outbreak were crowded living quarters, cold and moist weather, poor personal hygiene and improper sanitation [12]. It was also reported that humans became infected by eating infected birds, by poor hygiene procedures when cooking infected birds, or by close contact with infected poultry [13]. Therefore, sanitation is a core concept for preventive control of bird flu.

Human infection of H5N1 is a accepted as new emerging infectious disease. Most infected subjects have the history of contact with sick animals [14 – 17]. The patients commonly presented with presented with fever and respiratory symptoms [14 – 15]. Thorson et al recently done a research to analyze the association between flulike illness, defined as cough and fever, and exposure to sick or dead infected animals [16]. Thorson et al found that epidemiological data were concordant to transmission of mild, highly pathogenic avian influenza to humans and suggested that transmission could be more common than anticipated, although close contact seemed needed [16]. They noted that further microbiological investigations were indicated to validate these findings [16]. To evaluate risk factors for human infection with influenza A subtype H5N1, Dinh et al performed another well designed case-control study in Vietnam [18]. They noted that factors not associated with bird flu infection included raising healthy poultry, preparing healthy poultry for consumption, and exposure to persons with an acute respiratory illness [18]. Vong et al done another retrospective survey of poultry deaths and a seroepidemiologic investigation in a village where a 28-year-old man was reported for infection with H5N1 virus in March 2005 [19]. Despite frequent, direct contact with poultry suspected of having H5N1 virus infection, none of studied participants from all households had neutralizing antibodies to H5N1 [19]. Vong et al said that H5N1 virus transmission from poultry to humans remained low in this specific setting and bring a query for other possible mode of transmission of H5N1 [19]. In 2005, Ungchusak et al investigated possible person-to-person transmission in a family cluster of the bird flu infection in Thailand [20]. The index patient became ill three to four days after her last contact to dying household chickens [20]. Her mother came from a far city to care for this patient in the hospital, had no recognized exposure to animal, and later died from pneumonia [20]. The aunt also gave unprotected nursing care; she had fever five days after the mother first had fever, followed by pneumonia a week later [20]. Of interest, autopsy tissue from the mother and nasopharyngeal and throat swabs from the aunt were positive for H5N1 [20]. Ungchusak et al concluded that disease in the mother and aunt probably resulted from person-to-person transmission of this emerging influenza virus during unprotected exposure to the critically ill index patient [20].

How Can Bird Flu Become an Emerging Infectious Disease?

Bird flu, by its name, is the influenza virus infection of the bird or avian. The epidemic among the birds is not unusual. However, the outbreaks in other non avian species is of focused in the present day. These episodes seems to be problematic and brings attention from scientist around the world. "How can bird flu occurs in non avian species?" and "How can non avian species be infected?" are the two main questions in the present day. There are many theories to explain the findings. The first described hypothesis is the mutation of the virus. H5N1 is the virus among bird species that brings bird flu. The mutated H5N1 is widely mentioned. Indeed, any virus can be mutated in the environment. High rate of virus mutation can be expected. For further explanation, the author hereby will present the small bioinformatics research on this area in the following part in this chapter. However, due to the nature of virus, the high rate of mutation cannot be rejected. This is the fact but there has never been any reported problem. Therefore, if the mutated virus causes the epidemic is still a big query. Mutated H5N1 can be existed but it might not the cause of epidemic. Any virus can be mutated but it usually non sense. In addition, due to the existed literature, there has been no reported on sense mutation for isolated H5N1 around the world. The new non H5N1 mutated from classical H5N1 has never been documented. The clue for the story must be the others. The reassortment between influenza viruses is mentioned. However, until present, there is no existed evidence that there is reassortment between human influenza virus and bird influenza virus. In addition, reasssorment of viruses seems to be a very difficult process. The infection of the two kinds of influenza in the same situation is hardly to be seen. There several attempts to develop multiplex PCR for detection of co-infection of human influenza virus and bird influenza virus. This is not useful and not effective. Based on the fact that there is no chance for co-infection, no confirmed report, such diagnostic test seems to be useless and helpless. The low possibility of co-infection prevents this theory to be confirmed. The last theory is the explanation by host defect. Defect on host is possible. Some human hosts might have defect in the receptor that can receive the H5N1 virus. There is evidence confirming this proposal. Identification of receptor in reported infected host is documented. Whether general human beings pose this receptor is still be unknown and requires further research for confirmation.

The described processes are on the pathogenesis of bird flu. The emergence of infection has to be more focused. Bird is believed to be the problematic infected host transmitted disease to human beings. Birds can flu and the distance of flight is usually long. Some birds fly transcontinentally from cold to warm area. If infected bird fly in this migration, disease carrying to new settings can be expected. This is a high risk fact at present. However, the problem can lead more eminence in bird flu scenario than the mosquito borne infection which flies shorter distance. Infected bird flies and brings virus to new settings. If the condition is good, infection can be occurred. Usually, the pathogenesis of infection is very hard as already described. The problematic cases are usually the cases with confirmed history of contact with death corpses. The death chicken are usually documented in report. The died infected birds can also be eaten by local people with poor sanitation and this is questionable for transmission of infection. It is confirmed that eating is not the route of transmission but the contact with dead corpse is the cause. Direct contact must be avoided. Food sanitation is still necessary. Avoid contact death chicken and do not use it for cooking food is the basic rule. In addition, it should be mentioned for some risk rooted behavior among local population. Some people are closely contact to the bird in their family and can be the high risk for bird flu transmission.

Bird Flu Infection in India

As previously noted, bird flu is the new emerging infectious disease of the world. It is widely focused by medical scientist around the world. Although there is no specific report on human bird flu infection in India there are some interesting reports concerning bird flu from in India. The details are presented in Table 1.

In India, although there is no human infected case report. However, the existence of H5N1 in chicken imply high risk for possible new emerging of bird flu among local people. Indeed, chicken is the main meat for India, where the people mainly believe in Hinduism, which indicated no ingestion of beef. The problem of gastrointestinal infectious disease is common in India and the fact is due to the poor sanitation. Poor sanitation can be the problem that leading to the emerging of bird flu. If there is no good protocol to treat with the chicken meat, the problem can be occurred. The good management of food is acceptable protocol for control of bird flu in India.

Table 1. Reports on emerging bird flu infection in India.

Authors	Details
Rao [21]	Rao reported on modeling the rapid spread of avian influenza (H5N1) in India [21].
Tosh et al [22]	Tosh et al reported their genetic analysis of H9N2 avian influenza viruses isolated from India [22].
Murugkar et al [23]	Murugkar et al reported on H5N1 virus outbreaks in poultry in India [23].
Ray et al [24]	Ray et al reported on characterization of the complete genome of influenza A (H5N1) virus isolated during the 2006 outbreak in poultry in India [24].
CDC [25]	Outbreak news of avian influenza, India was reported [25].
Rao et al [26]	Rao et al reported on the results of isolation of variant influenza types A (H3N2), A (H1N1) and B strains in Pune, India [26].
Rao and Kadam [27]	Rao and Kadam reported on the results of isolation of recent variant influenza types A (H3N2) and B strains in Pune, India during 1998 [27].
Chakraborti [28]	Chakraborti discussed on pandemic management and developing world bioethics based on scenario of bird flu in Wes Bengal, India [28].

Analysis for Weak Linkage Prone for Mutation in Bird Flu Hemagglutinin

Presently, prediction of protein nanostructure and function is a modern way in studying by the proteomics and structural genomics era. To identify the point vulnerable to mutate is a new trend to expand the knowledge on disorders in genomic and proteomic level of several kinds of infectious diseases [29 - 30]. Generally, disordered regions in proteins often contain short linear peptide motifs that are important for protein function. Identification of the peptide motifs in the amino acid sequence can provide a good prediction for the weak linkages in a focused protein [29 - 30]. Here, the author performed a bioinformatic analysis to study the determine positions that trend to comply peptide motifs in the amino acid sequence of bird flu (H5N1) hemagglutinin. The database ExPASY [31] was selected as a tool and used for searching for the amino acid sequence of H5N1 hemagglutinin. Then the derived sequences from primary searching were used for further study on weak linkage. To find the weak linkage in H5N1 hemagglutinin, another computational bioinformatic tool namely GlobPlot [32] was applied. Basically, GlobPlot is a web service that permits the medical scientist to plot the tendency within the query protein for order/globularity and disorder [32]. It successfully find inter-domain segments containing linear motifs, as well as apparently ordered regions that have not any recognised domain [32]. In this work, H5N1 hemagglutinin (A/Pheasant/Hong Kong/FY155/01 (H5N1)) was used for further study. For this H5N1 hemagglutinin, there are 68 positions identified in this study. The identified positions are presented in Figure 1. The positions 91-100, 128-142, 279-301, 350-369 are identified as the position resist to mutation.

slvksdqici gyhannsteq vdtimeknvt vthaqdilek thngklcdld gvkplilrdc svagwllgnp mcdefinvpe wsyivekasp ANDLCYPGDF ndyeelkhll srinhfekiq iipksswSNH EASSGVSSAC PYlgkssffr nvv wlikknn ayptikrsyn ntnqedllvl wgihhpndaa eqtklyqnpt tyisvgtstl nqrlvpkiat rskvngqsgr meffwtilkp ndainfesng nfiapeyayk ivkkgdsaim kseleygnCN TKCQTPMGAI NSSMPFHNIH Pltigecpky vksnrlvlat glrntpqrer rrkkrglfga iagfieggwQ GMVDGWYGYH HSNEQGSGYa adkestqkai dgvtnkvnsi idkmntqfea vgrefnnler rienlnkkme dgfldvwtyn aellvlmene rtldfhdsnv knlydkvrlq lrdnakelgn gcfefyhkcd necmesvkng tydypqylrk aglnreeisg vklesmgtyq ilsiystvas slalaimvag lslwmcsngs lqcrici

Figure 1. Identified positions (in capital) that comply peptide motifs peptide motifs in amino acid sequence of H5N1 hemagglutinin.

Mutation of the virus is noted to be an important factor that can bring the pandemic of bird flu. Trampuz et al said that the widespread epidemic of bird flu in animals increases the likelihood for mutational scenarios and genetic reassortment [33]. Monitoring of mutational events turns to an important measure for infection control of bird flu [33 -34]. In many infectious diseases, the structural aberration in genome level is believed to be the major underlying pathiogenesis. Some disorders are mentioned as a single substitution with other effects on the sequence frame, the others are noted as a frameshift. The mutations in H5N1 hemagglutinin are noted to be the possible starting point for further pandemic of bird flu. Here, the author applies an algorithm to find the position in the amino acid sequences of H5N1 hemagglutinin that can be mutated. Here, the author can identify many positions. Some are already documented positions and the others has never been known. Here, it can be demonstrated that a simple diagnostic test for a single known mutation within H5N1 hemagglutinin cannot be the solution for successful in controlling of bird flu infection. Also, it might imply the probability for the occurrence of new escape mutant that cannot be detected by present standard PCR test. Based on this study, the weak linkages in the H5N1 hemagglutinin can be searched and can be good information for expectation of possible new mutations that can bring pandemic of H5N1 infection. In addition, the results from this study can be good information for further work on the diagnosis for mutants bird flu and vaccine development.

Oseltamivir for Treatment of Bird Flu

Oseltamivir is the first line drug for treatment of human bird flu.Pharmacologically, oseltamivir is a selective inhibitor of influenza A and B viral neuraminidase [35 – 37]. After absorption from the gastrointestinal tract oseltamivir is efficiently converted to GS4071, which is persisted at high and sustained concentrations in plasma [35 – 40]. Oral oseltamivir was an effective treatment in naturally occurring influenza when administered within 3 days of symptom onset, minimizing both the duration and severity of symptoms and the incidence of secondary complications in influenza-infected patients enrolled in 2 large placebo-controlled, double-blind trials [35 – 40]. The major manufacturer of oseltamivir is Roche company and the commercial name is "Tamiflu R" . Generally, there are two main forms of Tamiflu, capsule (75 mg) and powder. Tamiflu can be well absorbed in the gastrointestinal tract and further metabolized at liver into the active form, oseltamivir carboxylate. The oseltamivir carboxylate can actively get rid of the virus and has a half life about 6-10 hours. It is excreted via kidney, therefore, it is needed to modify dosage in the case with renal impairment. This drug is also presently use for treatment and prevention of bird flu.

References

[1] Kiselev OI, Sominina AA, Grinbaum EB. Influenza: current status and epidemiologic situation. *Vestn Ross Akad Med Nauk*. 1994;(9):3-7.

[2] Hosrtmann DM. Clinical virology. *Am J Med*. 1965 May;38:738-50.

[3] Skehel JJ, Wiley DC. Influenza viruses and cell membranes. *Am J Respir Crit Care Med*. 1995 Oct;152(4 Pt 2):S13-5.

[4] Nayak DP, Hui EK, Barman S. Assembly and budding of influenza virus. *Virus Res*. 2004 Dec;106(2):147-65.

[5] Schmitt AP, Lamb RA. Escaping from the cell: assembly and budding of negative-strand RNA viruses. *Curr Top Microbiol Immunol*. 2004;283:145-96.

[6] Day T, Andre JB, Park A. The evolutionary emergence of pandemic influenza. *Proc Biol Sci*. 2006 Dec 7;273(1604):2945-53.

[7] Bergner L, Yerby AS. Low income and barriers to use of health services. *N Engl J Med*. 1968 Mar 7;278(10):541-6.

[8] Killingray D. The influenza pandemic of 1918-1919 in the British Caribbean. *Soc Hist Med*. 1994 Apr;7(1):59-87.

[9] Ompad DC, Galea S, Blaney S, Coady MH, Sisco S, Glidden K, Vlahov D. Access to influenza vaccine in East Harlem and the Bronx during a national vaccine shortage. *J Community Health*. 2007 Jun;32(3):195-202.

[10] Cristalli A, Capua I. Practical problems in controlling H5N1 high pathogenicity avian influenza at village level in Vietnam and introduction of biosecurity measures. *Avian* Dis. 2007 Mar;51(1 Suppl):461-2.

[11] Ferguson N. Poverty, death, and a future influenza pandemic. *Lancet*. 2006 Dec 23;368(9554):2187-8.

[12] Tangkanakul W, Tharmaphornpilas P, Thawatsupha P, Laolukpong P, Lertmongkol J. An outbreak of Influenza A virus in a hilltribe village of Mae Hong Son Province Thailand, 1997. *J Med Assoc Thai*. 2000 Sep;83(9):1005-10.

[13] Angelava NA, Angelava AV. Epidemiology, clinical picture, prevention and treatment of Avian influenza. *Georgian Med News*. 2006 Feb;(131):69-76.

[14] Tran TH, Nguyen TL, Nguyen TD, Luong TS, Pham PM, Nguyen VC, Pham TS, Vo CD, Le TQ, Ngo TT, Dao BK, Le PP, Nguyen TT, Hoang TL, Cao VT, Le TG, Nguyen DT, Le HN, Nguyen KT, Le HS, Le VT, Christiane D, Tran TT, Menno de J, Schultsz C, Cheng P, Lim W, Horby P, Farrar J; World Health Organization International Avian Influenza Investigative Team. Avian influenza A (H5N1) in 10 patients in Vietnam. *N Engl J Med.* 2004 Mar 18;350(12):1179-88.

[15] Chotpitayasunondh T, Ungchusak K, Hanshaoworakul W, Chunsuthiwat S, Sawanpanyalert P, Kijphati R, Lochindarat S, Srisan P, Suwan P, Osotthanakorn Y, Anantasetagoon T, Kanjanawasri S, Tanupattarachai S, Weerakul J, Chaiwirattana R, Maneerattanaporn M, Poolsavathitikool R, Chokephaibulkit K, Apisarnthanarak A, Dowell SF. Human disease from influenza A (H5N1), Thailand, 2004. *Emerg Infect Dis*. 2005 Feb;11(2):201-9.

[16] Thorson A, Petzold M, Nguyen TK, Ekdahl K. Is exposure to sick or dead poultry associated with flulike illness?: a population-based study from a rural area in Vietnam with outbreaks of highly pathogenic avian influenza. *Arch Intern Med.* 2006 Jan 9;166(1):119-23.

[17] Groome PA, Richardson H. Flulike illness and exposure to sick or dead poultry. Arch *Intern Med.* 2006 Jul 10;166(13):1420-1.

[18] Dinh PN, Long HT, Tien NT, Hien NT, Mai le TQ, Phong le H, Tuan le V, Van Tan H, Nguyen NB, Van Tu P, Phuong NT; World Health Organization/Global Outbreak Alert and Response Network Avian Influenza Investigation Team in Vietnam. Risk factors for human infection with avian influenza A H5N1, Vietnam, 2004. *Emerg Infect Dis.* 2006 Dec;12(12):1841-7.

[19] Vong S, Coghlan B, Mardy S, Holl D, Seng H, Ly S, Miller MJ, Buchy P, Froehlich Y, Dufourcq JB, Uyeki TM, Lim W, Sok T. Low frequency of poultry-to-human H5NI virus transmission, southern Cambodia, 2005. *Emerg Infect Dis.* 2006 Oct;12(10):1542-7.

[20] Ungchusak K, Auewarakul P, Dowell SF, Kitphati R, Auwanit W, Puthavathana P, Uiprasertkul M, Boonnak K, Pittayawonganon C, Cox NJ, Zaki SR, Thawatsupha P, Chittaganpitch M, Khontong R, Simmerman JM, Chunsutthiwat S. Probable person-to-person transmission of avian influenza A (H5N1). *N Engl J Med.* 2005 Jan 27;352(4):333-40.

[21] Rao AS. Modeling the rapid spread of avian influenza (h5n1) in India.Math Biosci Eng. 2008 Jul;5(3):523-37.

[22] Tosh C, Nagarajan S, Behera P, Rajukumar K, Purohit K, Kamal RP, Murugkar HV, Gounalan S, Pattnaik B, Vanamayya PR, Pradhan HK, Dubey SC. Genetic analysis of H9N2 avian influenza viruses isolated from India.

[23] Murugkar HV, Nagarajan S, Tosh C, Bhatia S, Venkatesh G, Jain R, Kumar S, Khandia R, Pandey M, Behera P, Tripathy S, Kulkarni DD, Dubey SC. H5N1 virus outbreaks in poultry in India. *Vet Rec.* 2008 Feb 23;162(8):255.

[24] Ray K, Potdar VA, Cherian SS, Pawar SD, Jadhav SM, Waregaonkar SR, Joshi AA, Mishra AC. Characterization of the complete genome of influenza A (H5N1) virus isolated during the 2006 outbreak in poultry in India. *Virus Genes.* 2008 Apr;36(2):345-53

[25] Outbreak news. Avian influenza, India. *Wkly Epidemiol Rec.* 2006 Feb 24;81(8):70.

[26] Rao BL, Kadam SS, Pawar MS. Isolation of recent variant influenza types A(H3N2), A (H1N1) & B strains in Pune, India. *Indian J Med Res.* 2001 Nov;114:157-9.

[27] Rao BL, Kadam SS. Isolation of recent variant influenza types A (H3N2) & B strains in Pune, India during 1998. *Indian J Med Res.* 2000 Jan;111:3-5.

[28] Chakraborti C. Pandemic management and developing world bioethics: bird flu in Wes Bengal. *Dev World Bioeth.* 2008 Aug 11. [Epub ahead of print]

[29] Lee C, Wang Q. Bioinformatics analysis of alternative splicing. *Brief Bioinform* 2005;6:23-33.

[30] Levin JM, Penland RC, Stamps AT, Cho CR. Using in silico biology to facilitate drug development. *Novartis Found Symp* 2002;247:222-38.

[31] Gasteiger E, Gattiker A, Hoogland C, Ivanyi I, Appel RD, Bairoch A. ExPASy: The proteomics server for in-depth protein knowledge and analysis. *Nucleic Acids Res.* 2003;31:3784-8.

[32] Linding R, Russell RB, Neduva V, Gibson TJ. GlobPlot: Exploring protein sequences for globularity and disorder. *Nucleic Acids Res* 2003 ;31:3701-8.

[33] Prabhu RM Avian influenza: a new pandemic threat? *Mayo Clin Proc.* 2004;79:523-30.

[34] Keawchareon J, Oraveerakul K, Poovorawan. The genome sequence analysis of H5N1 avian influenza A virus isolated from the outbreak among poultry populations in Thailand. *Virology.* 2004;328:169-76.

[35] Schunemann HJ, Hill SR, Kakad M, Bellamy R, Uyeki TM, Hayden FG, Yazdanpanah Y, Beigel J, Chotpitayasunondh T, Del Mar C, Farrar J, Tran TH, Ozbay B, Sugaya N, Fukuda K, Shindo N, Stockman L, Vist GE, Croisier A, Nagjdaliyev A, Roth C, Thomson G, Zucker H, Oxman AD; WHO Rapid Advice Guideline Panel on Avian Influenza. WHO Rapid Advice Guidelines for pharmacological management of sporadic human infection with avian influenza A (H5N1) virus. *Lancet Infect Dis.* 2007 Jan;7(1):21-31.

[36] Bardsley-Elliot A, Noble S. Oseltamivir. *Drugs.* 1999 Nov;58(5):851-60.

[37] McClellan K, Perry CM. Oseltamivir: a review of its use in influenza. *Drugs.* 2001;61(2):263-83.

[38] McNicholl IR, McNicholl JJ. Neuraminidase inhibitors: zanamivir and oseltamivir. *Ann Pharmacother.* 2001 Jan;35(1):57-70.

[39] Hayden FG, Treanor JJ, Fritz RS, Lobo M, Betts RF, Miller M, Kinnersley N, Mills RG, Ward P, Straus SE. Use of the oral neuraminidase inhibitor oseltamivir in experimental human influenza: randomized controlled trials for prevention and treatment. *JAMA.* 1999 Oct 6;282(13):1240-6.

[40] Treanor JJ, Hayden FG, Vrooman PS, Barbarash R, Bettis R, Riff D, Singh S, Kinnersley N, Ward P, Mills RG. Efficacy and safety of the oral neuraminidase inhibitor oseltamivir in treating acute influenza: a randomized controlled trial. US Oral Neuraminidase Study Group. *JAMA.* 2000 Feb 23;283(8):1016-24.

Chapter XV

Scrub Typhus in India

Introduction to Scrub Typhus [1 - 20]

Scrub typhus by definition is an infection caused by rickettsial pathogen, *Orientia tsutsugamushi*. The pathogen, an obligate intracellular bacterium, was firstly isolated in 1930. There are many possible infections due to rickettsia in medicine. The rickettsial infection can be seen elsewhere around the world. However, scrub typhus is the rickettsial infection that is common in the tropical regions. This might be due to the nature of the pathogen and the abundance of insect vector in this area. Scrub typhus is a vector borne disease. The tick is the vector for this infection. Scrub typhus is endemic in Asia. Local people's behavior and climatic changes can influence the occurrence of the disease. Concerning the nature of vector borne disease, it relates strongly to the poverty as well as climate. Poverty means poor and this prevents good sanitation. Insect vector is more prevalent in the places with poor sanitation. This is also the places for the poor. India has millions of the poor, therefore, abundance of vectors can be expected. Focusing on the climate, the hot monsoon type climate helps propagate of the insect vector and this is the actual climate of the tropical countries of Asia. Increasing prevalences of scrub typhus have been reported from some Asian countries and may accompany with the widespread use of beta-lactam antibiotics or to improve diagnostic tools [20].

Focusing of the clinical presentation, fever is common. However, this is not specific clinical manifestations. Other tropical infection as dengue fever, viral encephalitis, melioidosis, leptospirosis also have the main presentation as fever. Luckily, there is another pathognomomic presentation, a dermatological appearance namely eschar lesion. This is a specific skin lesion for this infection. It is concluded that scrub typhus should be considered in any febrile patient presenting with a macular rash, a polyadenopathy, an eschar, or a history of visiting to the endemic areas. Routinely, diagnosis of scrub typhus is based on the patient's history of exposure, clinical appearances, and results of serologic testing. Regional and generalized lymphadenopathy can be seen [21]. The pulmonary signs of scrub typhus include interstitial pneumonia, interstitial edema, and hemorrhage owing to vasculitis. Abdominal signs include splenomegaly, periportal edema, gallbladder wall thickening, and lymphadenopathy [21]. The diagnosis of scrub typhus using indirect immunofluorescence assay should be based on a level equal to or more than four-fold increase in the titer in paired serum samples or based on a single sample titer when there is a sufficient local evidence base [22]. However, the public health importance of this disease is underestimated owing to difficulties with clinical diagnosis and lack of laboratory methods in several endemic settings [7].

After confirmation of diagnosis, treatment with doxycycline or tetracycline should be used [16]. Panpanich and Garner noted that tetracycline and doxycycline was still effective in treating scrub typhus and further research was needed to identify appropriate treatment in areas where *Orientia tsutsugamushi* resistant to doxycycline has been reported [16]. Recent reports of scrub typhus outbreaks in endemic areas, and an increased antibiotic resistance implies a requirement for a suitable vaccine for scrub typhus. For prevention, disease surveillance program is suggested, and vector control programs must be organized in effective way.

Scrub Typhus Infection in India

As previously noted, scrub typhus infection can be classified as an important vector borne infection. India is a country facing up with the problem of many new infections and reappearances of infections. Scrub typhus infection in India is considered problematic to be focused. There are many reports on scrub typhus emerging in India. The summary of important reports is shown in Table 1.

Table 1. Reports on emerging scrub typhus infections in India.

Authors	Details
Kumar et al [23]	Kumar et al reported on an outbreak investigation of scrub in Himachal Pradesh, India [23]
Sharma et al [24]	Sharma et al performed an investigation of an outbreak of scrub typhus in the himalayan region of India [24].
Mathai et al [25]	Mathai et al reported on an outbreak of scrub typhus in southern India during the cooler months [25].

Scrub Typhus Infections in Other Countries in South Asia

Scrub typhus infection can also be seen in other countries in South Asia. However, there is no report on emerging or outbreak of this disease in other countries in South Asia. The main reason might be due to the limited source of insect vector in other countries.

References

[1] Botelho-Nevers E, Raoult D. Fever of unknown origin due to rickettsioses. *Infect Dis Clin North Am*. 2007 Dec;21(4):997-1011, ix.

[2] Lee KL, Lee JK, Yim YM, Lim OK, Bae KH. Acute transverse myelitis associated with scrub typhus: case report and a review of literatures. *Diagn Microbiol Infect Dis*. 2008 Feb;60(2):237-9.

[3] Tachibana N, Okayama A. Tsutsugamushi disease (scrub typhus). *Nippon Rinsho*. 2007 Mar 28;65 Suppl 3:208-11.

[4] Chattopadhyay S, Richards AL. Scrub typhus vaccines: past history and recent developments. *Hum Vaccin*. 2007 May-Jun;3(3):73-80.

[5] Mahara F. Rickettsioses in Japan and the far East. *Ann N Y Acad Sci*. 2006 Oct;1078:60-73

[6] Parola P, Raoult D. Tropical rickettsioses. *Clin Dermatol*. 2006 May-Jun;24(3):191-200.

[7] Mahajan SK. Scrub typhus. *J Assoc Physicians India*. 2005 Nov;53:954-8. Gupta V, Gautam V. Scrub Typhus--A short review. *J Commun Dis*. 2004 Dec;36(4):284-9.

[8] Amano K. Tsutsugamushi disease rickettsia. *Nippon Rinsho*. 2005 Jul;63 Suppl 7:231-3.

[9] Bernabeu-Wittel M, Segura-Porta F. Rickettsioses. *Enferm Infecc Microbiol Clin*. 2005 Mar;23(3):163-72.

[10] Jensenius M, Fournier PE, Raoult D. Rickettsioses and the international traveler. *Clin Infect Dis*. 2004 Nov 15;39(10):1493-9.

[11] Watt G, Parola P. Scrub typhus and tropical rickettsioses. *Curr Opin Infect Dis*. 2003 Oct;16(5):429-36.

[12] Yen TH, Chang CT, Lin JL, Jiang JR, Lee KF. Scrub typhus: a frequently overlooked cause of acute renal failure. *Ren Fail*. 2003 May;25(3):397-410.

[13] Tachibana N, Okayama A. Tsutsugamushi disease. *Nippon Rinsho*. 2003 Feb;61 Suppl 2:500-4.

[14] Oda H. Rickettsial diseases. *Nippon Rinsho*. 2001 Nov;59 Suppl 7:162-9.

[15] Kovácová E, Kazár J. Rickettsial diseases and their serological diagnosis. *Clin Lab*. 2000;46(5-6):239-45.

[16] Panpanich R, Garner P. Antibiotics for treating scrub typhus. *Cochrane Database Syst Rev*. 2000;(2):CD002150.

[17] Amano K. Orientia tsutsugamushi. *Nippon Rinsho*. 1999 Nov;57 Suppl:207-9.

[18] Tamura A. Microbiology of Orientia tsutsugamushi. *Nippon Saikingaku Zasshi*. 1999 Nov;54(4):815-32.

[19] Tachibana N. Classic type tsutsugamushi disease. *Ryoikibetsu Shokogun Shirizu*. 1999;(24 Pt 2):288-90.

[20] Silpapojakul K. Scrub typhus in the Western Pacific region. *Ann Acad Med Singapore*. 1997 Nov;26(6):794-800.

[21] Jeong YJ, Kim S, Wook YD, Lee JW, Kim KI, Lee SH. Scrub typhus: clinical, pathologic, and imaging findings. *Radiographics*. 2007 Jan-Feb;27(1):161-72.

[22] Blacksell SD, Bryant NJ, Paris DH, Doust JA, Sakoda Y, Day NP. Scrub typhus serologic testing with the indirect immunofluorescence method as a diagnostic gold standard: a lack of consensus leads to a lot of confusion. *Clin Infect Dis*. 2007 Feb 1;44(3):391-401.

[23] Kumar K, Saxena VK, Thomas TG, Lal S. Outbreak investigation of scrub Typhus in Himachal Pradesh (India). *J Commun Dis.* 2004 Dec;36(4):277-83.

[24] Sharma A, Mahajan S, Gupta ML, Kanga A, Sharma V. Investigation of an outbreak of scrub typhus in the himalayan region of India. *Jpn J Infect Dis.* 2005 Aug;58(4):208-10.

[25] Mathai E, Rolain JM, Verghese GM, Abraham OC, Mathai D, Mathai M, Raoult D. Outbreak of scrub typhus in southern India during the cooler months. *Ann N Y Acad Sci.* 2003 Jun;990:359-64

Chapter XVI

Buffalopox in India

Introduction to Buffalopox [1 - 6]

Mainly, outbreaks of buffalopox affect buffaloes, cows and humans in many parts of the world [1]. Since the first outbreak in India, a large number of epidemics are reported around the world [1]. This affects the dairy industry. Singh et al reported that the causative pathogen, buffalopox virus (BPXV), was a member of the Orthopoxvirus, and was closely related to Vaccinia virus (VACV), the type-species of the genus [1 - 2]. Tuner and Baxby observed that controlled degradation of virions showed that the polypeptides which enabled the viruses to be differentiated were located in the surface and sub-surface layers [3]. Tuner and Baxby noted that this might relate to the infectious property [3]. *Dumbell* and *Richardson* performed virological investigations of specimens from buffaloes affected by buffalopox in Maharashtra State, India between 1985 and 1987 [4]. In this work, isolates of poxviruses were made from specimens of scabs taken from pox lesions on buff [4]. *Dumbell* and *Richardson* found that the biological characters of most isolates resembled those of the Hissar strain of buffalopox virus, except for one isolate which appeared to be vaccinia [4]. They finally concluded that buffalopox was an emerging enzootic virus and was a subspecies of vaccinia virus [4]. Until present, continuous researches on this new emerging viruses are still undergone.

Considering the clinical appearance, dermatological manifestation is common.

In humans, pox lesions can be seen on the hands whereas in affected buffaloes and cows the lesions can be commonly detected majorly on the teats and udder [5]. For diagnosis, virus can be isolated from the skin scabs collected from infected humans and animals [1 – 6]. Viral isolation in Vero cell cultures and detection of viral nucleotide sequences by polymerase chain reaction (PCR) are useful for confirming the exact etiology of the disease [1 – 6]. Usually, cases of human infection are seen particularly in milkers working with the affected herds. Singh et al said that infected milkers usually develope pox-like lesions on the skin of the hands, forearms and forehead accompanied by fever for three days, axillary lymphadenopathy and general malaise [6]. I

Table 1. Reports on new studies on virology of buffalopox virus.

Authors	Details
Singh et al [7]	Singh et al reported on sequence analysis of C18L gene of buffalopox virus as PCR strategy for specific detection and differentiation of buffalopox from orthopoxviruses [7].
Ciulla et al [8]	Ciulla et al reported on evolutionary history of orthopoxvirus proteins similar to human complement regulators [8].
Anand Kumar and Butchaiah [9]	Anand Kumar and Butchaiah reported on partial antigenic characterization of buffalopox virus [9].
Ropp et al [10]	Ropp et al reported on PCR strategy for identification and differentiation of small pox and other orthopoxviruses [10].
Hill et al [11]	Hill et al reported on microelectrophoresis of enzyme and chemically treated viruses and cores of vaccinia, buffalopox, variola and alastrim [11].

Buffalo Pox Infection in India

As previously noted, buffalopox outbreak was firstly reported from India. This is classified as the actual new emerging infectious disease of India. There are some interesting reports on emerging of this disease in India. The details are presented in Table 2.

Table 2. Reports on emerging buffalopox infection in India.

Authors	Details
Kolhapure et al [5]	Kolhapure et al reported an investigation of buffalopox outbreaks in Maharashtra State during 1992-1996 [5].
Singh et al [6]	Singh et al reported on an outbreak of buffalopox in buffalo dairy herds in Aurangabad, India [6].

The effect of buffalopox infection in social aspect must be said. Due to the panic of the disease, similar to other outbreak, the milk consumption after the news of outbreak usually significantly reduced implying the effect on dairy economy. To cope with the specific outbreak, education to the local population might be the helpful to relieve the panic.

References

[1] Singh RK, Hosamani M, Balamurugan V, Bhanuprakash V, Rasool TJ, Yadav MP. Buffalopox: an emerging and re-emerging zoonosis. *Anim Health Res Rev.* 2007 Jun;8(1):105-14.

[2] Lal SM, Singh IP. Buffalopox-a review. *Trop Anim Health Prod.* 1977 May;9(2):107-12

[3] Turner A, Baxby D. Structural polypeptides of Orthopoxvirus: their distribution in various members and location within the virion. *J Gen Virol.* 1979 Dec;45(3):537-45.

[4] Dumbell K, Richardson M. Virological investigations of specimens from buffaloes affected by buffalopox in Maharashtra State, India between 1985 and 1987. *Arch Virol.* 1993;128(3-4):257-67.

[5] Kolhapure RM, Deolankar RP, Tupe CD, Raut CG, Basu A, Dama BM, Pawar SD, Joshi MV, Padbidri VS, Goverdhan MK, Banerjee K. Investigation of buffalopox outbreaks in Maharashtra State during 1992-1996. *Indian J Med Res.* 1997 Nov;106:441-6.

[6] Singh RK, Hosamani M, Balamurugan V, Satheesh CC, Shingal KR, Tatwarti SB, Bambal RG, Ramteke V, Yadav MP. An outbreak of buffalopox in buffalo (Bubalus bubalis) dairy herds in Aurangabad, *India. Rev Sci Tech.* 2006 Dec;25(3):981-7.

[7] Singh RK, Balamurugan V, Hosamani M, Kallesh DJ, Bhanuprakash V. Sequence analysis of C18L gene of buffalopox virus: PCR strategy for specific detection and differentiation of buffalopox from orthopoxviruses. *J Virol Methods.* 2008 Sep 11. [Epub ahead of print]

[8] Ciulla E, Emery A, Konz D, Krushkal J. Evolutionary history of orthopoxvirus proteins similar to human complement regulators. *Gene.* 2005 Aug 1;355:40-7.

[9] Anand Kumar P, Butchaiah G. Partial antigenic characterization of buffalopox virus. *Vet Res Commun.* 2004 Aug;28(6):543-52.

[10] Ropp SL, Jin Q, Knight JC, Massung RF, Esposito JJ. PCR strategy for identification and differentiation of small pox and other orthopoxviruses. *J Clin Microbiol.* 1995 Aug;33(8):2069-76.

[11] Hill BJ, Baxby D, Douglas HW. Microelectrophoresis of enzyme and chemically treated viruses and cores of vaccinia, buffalopox, variola and alastrim. *J Gen Virol.* 1972 Jul;16(1):39-46.

Chapter XVII

HIV and Related Emerging Infections in India

Introduction to HIV [1 - 10]

Human immunodeficiency virus or HIV infection is a very well known viral infection in the present day. This is defined as a new emerging viral infection in the past 2 decades. At this time, this is not an emerging infection. However, it is associated with other relating emerging infections. Those infections are due to the immunodeficiency stage in the HIV infected cases. At the time of discovery, the impaired immune status is the presentation of affected cases. This is a mysterious for a long time. After the succeed in identification of HIV virus, this disease became well known and accepted as the most important immunodeficiency syndrome. HIV is accepted as the pathogenic organism. Indeed, HIV infection seems to be a complex disease. There are many researches and developments for HIV. There is also specific branch of medicine called HIV medicine. The knowledge on HIV infection is required for all physicians at present.

Focusing on the pathogenesis of HIV, the HIV is a retrovirus. It directly infected CD4+ T lymphocytes, hence, cellular immunity is primary affected. There are several modes of transmission for HIV. However, the three important modes are 1) sexually transmission (both homosexual and heterosexual cases), 2) blood and blood products transmission and c) transmission via sharing of needle for intravenous injection. At first, the cases are seen in those with homosexual behavior and intravenous drug users. Later, it came to hit the heterosexual group, husband and wife infection. The blooming of the HIV infection occurred at this time. Later, the HIV infection became the problem for the newborns, who were the child to HIV infected mothers. It can be said that HIV infection hits the whole family. The disease becomes one of the most important infectious diseases at present day.

There is no curative treatment for this disease. There are many newly developed antiretroviral drugs that can inactivate but not cure the disease. For diagnosis, there are several diagnostic tools for HIV. However, thousands of techniques still have their limitation. This is the basic concept of laboratory medicine that there is no best test for all scenarios. It can be said that HIV infection becomes problem for all countries around the world. Many infectious diseases relating to HIV become emerging. New emerging and reemerging infections related to HIV infection are noted in medicine. These conditions include opportunistic infection as well as antiretroviral drug resistant HIV. In this chapter, the details of these important problems will be detailed.

Antiretroviral Drug Resistant HIV Infection in India

Antiretroviral resistant HIV infection is the HIV infection that is resistant to antiretroviral drug. This condition contributed to the problematic HIV infectious cases. Antiretroviral resistant HIV infection is emerging as one of the most problematic infectious disease in medical history [11 - 20]. It is noted to be created by medical personnel who administer antiretroviral drugs improperly. The diagnosis for antiretroviral drug resistant is the new laboratory investigation for management of HIV infected cases with the problem of response to standard antiretroviral regimen. This problem is also observed in India and is still the present problem. Some important reports are presented in Table 1.

Table 1. Reports on Antiretroviral drug resistant HIV infections in India.

Author	Details
Sachdeva et al [21]	Sachdeva et al reported on incidence of lamivudine resistance associated mutations in pol-gene of HIV-1 in patients from north India [21].
Pachamuthu et al [22]	Pachamuthu et al reported and discussed on HIV-1 drug resistance among untreated patients in India [22].
Saple et al [23]	Saple et al mentioned for the difficulties encountered with the use of antiretroviral drugs in India [23].
Nagelkerke et al [24]	Nagelkerke et al reported on modelling HIV/AIDS epidemics in Botswana and India focusing impact of interventions to prevent transmission [24].
Kumarasamy et al [25]	Kumarasamy et al reported on the usage of antiretroviral drugs in the treatment of people living with HIV infection in a south Indian tertiary referral centre [25].

Important mutations in HIV-1 reverse transcriptase: an explanation in nanostructure level based on the view of energy change

1. Introduction

HIV infection is an important infection affecting a million of world population. Until present, developement of a prophylactic vaccine for HIV-1 is not successful. Despite two decades of effort, it is still a long way off [26]. The best present way in coping with the patients with HIV infection is controlling of disease with antiretroviral drugs. However, a new emerging problem of antiretroviral drug usage is the problem of drug resistance. Standardized surveillance of transmitted and treatment-associated HIV drug resistance is very important to the success of antiretroviral therapy expansion in developing countries [27]. Routine assessment of prescribing practices, availability of and access to proper medical regimens for adults and children, antiretroviral drug supply continuity, and means to prevent HIV transmission will supply very important information for HIV drug-resistance prevention [27]. DNA polymerase and RNase H activities of HIV reverse transcriptase (RT) have been mentioned as potential targets for antiretroviral therapy for many years [28]. The development of medicines targeting the DNA polymerase activity has been highly successful, with presently more than ten drugs approved for the treatment of HIV infection and more alternatives in preclinical and clinical development [28]. However, the drug resistance owing to the mutation of HIV-RT becomes a new interesting problem in HIV medicine.

Mutations at either Tyr181 or Tyr188 within HIV-1 reverse transcriptase (RT) give high level resistance to many first generation non-nucleoside inhibitors (NNRTIs) such as the anti-AIDS drug nevirapine. Lys103Asn and Tyr181Cys are the two mutations frequently observed in patients exposed to various non-nucleoside reverse transcriptase inhibitor drugs (NNRTIs) [29]. HIV strains containing both reverse transcriptase (RT) mutations are highly resistant to all of the approved NNRTI drugs [29]. However, the exact nature in nanostructure level of the effect of such mutations has never been completely mentioned and this can be important data for further implication in the HIV-RT mutants related antiretroviral drug resistance. In this work, the author simulated for the required energy corresponding to the mentioned two important mutations of HIV-RT. This study can provide an explanation in nanostructure level based on the view of energy change.

2. Materials and Methods

2.1. Basic Concepts in Reaction between Antiretroviral Drug and HIV-RT

As previously mentioned, DNA polymerase and RNase H activities of HIV-RT is the major target for antiretroviral drug. In this work, the author selected to studied the two most important mutants for HIV-RT, Lys103Asn and Tyr181Cys. Further evaluation for the energy change in these two focused mutations were performed.

2.2. Quantum Chemical Analysis for Bonding Energy

This is a calculation - based work. The quantum chemical analysis for the whole reaction was performed according to the classical bonding theory [29]. Basically, each chemical reaction poses it specific required reaction energy. The primary assumption in this study is that the required reaction energy for the pharmacological reaction between antiretroviral drug and HIV-RT is equal to "A" kCal/mol for one mole of resulted complex and this parameter is accepted as a constant parameter. The net energy requirement in kCal for a reaction relies on the amount of two substrates, one mole of antiretroviral drug and one mole of HIV-RT. Here, another primary assumption is that the amount of the two substrates is equal to "B" g and "C" g for antiretroviral drug and HIV-RT in general reaction with wild type of HIV-RT.

However, the significant change in the mutants of HIV-RT is the amino acid, which impacts the amount of the substrate HIV-RT. In this work, the theoretical simulation for the two studied mutants was performed. Calculation for the amount of HIV-RT in each mutant was performed. Further calculation for the net energy requirement for a reaction was finally done.

3. Results

For the Lys103Asn mutant, the main change is Lys (weight = 146.19 g/mol) to Asn (weight = 132.12 g/mol). The chaning in molecular weight due to this mutant and its corresponding net energy requirement are calculated and presented in Table 1.For the Tyr181Cys mutant, the main change is Tyr (weight = 181.19 g/mol) to Cys (weight = 121.16 g/mol). The changing in molecular weight due to this mutant and its corresponding net energy requirement are calculated and presented in Table 2. The net energy requirements are most Tyr181Cys mutant in and least in wild type.

Table 2. Change in amount of HIV-RT and net energy requirement for Lys103Asn and Tyr181Cys mutants HIV-1 RT.

HIV-RT types	Amount (g)	Net energy requirement* (kCal/mol)
Wild	C	A/C
Lys103Asn mutant	C-146.19 +132.12	A/C-14.07
Tyr181Cys mutant	C-181.19 +121.16	A/C-60.07

* compared to one mole of substrate HIV-RT

4. Discussion

Inhibitors of HIV reverse transcriptase (RT) are important drugs for the treatment of AIDS [30]. Numerous potent inhibitors of RT have been described including all of the drugs that have been presently licensed for the treatment of AIDS, but their efficacy has been blocked by the emergence of drug-resistant HIV variants [31]. The HIV viral resistance to the compounds may arise through different mutations, depending on the nature of the compounds and the group to which they belong [32].Extensive biochemical, genetic, and clinical data about HIV-RT enzymatic mechanisms, inhibition, and drug resistance have been mentioned [31].

HIV-RT mutants confer high levels of HIV resistance to antiviral drugs [32]. However, while conferring drug resistance, they can also reduce viral replication capacity [32]. The molecular mechanisms behind remain mainly unknown. Recently, Das et al studied the crystal structures of Lys103Asn and Tyr181Cys mutants HIV-1 RT and found that NNRTIs restricted the flexibility of the YMDD loop and inhibited the catalytic aspartate residues from adopting their metal-binding conformations [29]. In this theoretical research, the author tried to explain the energy change corresponding to the focused mutations within HIV-RT. Here, the author found that both mutants critically impact the net energy requirement. Increased energy requirement can be detected. This implies the difficulties for occurrence of reaction and further means the drug resistance. Based on the results in this study, it seems that Tyr181Cys mutant might pose more drug resistance property than Lys103Asn mutant. The results from this study can be useful for future antiretroviral drug design and coping with the problem of HIV-RT related drug resistance.

Problems of Opportunistic Infections in India

As already mentioned, opportunistic infection becomes new problems in infectious medicine in the era of HIV infection. There are several kinds of opportunistic infections in HIV. The important details of important opportunistic infection, which can cause outbreak, in HIV infected patients in India will be hereby summarized and presented.

1. Tuberculosis

Tuberculosis is an important opportunistic infection in HIV infected patients. There are many reports confirming the reemerging of tuberculosis in India in the era of HIV epidemics. More details can be seen in another separated chapter in this book.

2. Cryptosporidiosis [33 – 42]

Cryptosporidiosis is an important opportunistic protozoa infection. This is the focused opportunistic protozonal infection in the present day. By nature, the cryptosporidiosis is classified as a water borne disease and can be the cause of outbreak. The direct threat of contaminated water to human is not too much due to the fact that most contaminated water samples are not normal drinking water but water in river or canal. However, the problem generally occurs due to further contamination in bivalve shellfish in the seashore where the contaminated water is collected. This problem is also observed in India and is still the present problem. Some important reports are presented in Table 3.

3. Toxoplasmosis [47 – 55]

Toxoplasmosis is generated by *Toxoplasma gondii*, a protozoan parasite that infects up to a third of the world's population [47 - 55]. Infection is commonly acquired by ingestion of food that is contaminated with oocysts. Neurolopical manifestation of toxoplasmosis can be fatal. This can cause seizure as well as increased intracranial pressure. The diagnosis by imaging technology is useful. The ring like lesion from CT brain in HIV infected cases is the pathogenomonic feature. This infection is a member of TORCH agent which can cause congenital anomaly. For sure, it is the big problem for the pregnant with HIV infection. There are some reports on toxoplasmosis outbreak in India [56]. This problem is also important problem of HIV infected cases in India [57].

Table 3. Reports on the emergence of cryptosporidiosis in HIV infection in India.

Author	Details
Kaushik et al [43]	Kaushik et al performed an evaluation of staining techniques, antigen detection and nested PCR for the diagnosis of cryptosporidiosis in HIV seropositive and seronegative patients [43].
Jayalakshmi et al [44]	Jayalakshmi et al performed an evaluation of an enzyme-linked immunoassay for the detection of Cryptosporidium antigen in fecal specimens of HIV/AIDS patients [44].
Rao Ajjampur et al [45]	Rao Ajjampur et al described for clinical features and risk factors associated with cryptosporidiosis in HIV infected adults in India [45].
Muthusamy et al [46]	Muthusamy et al reported on multilocus genotyping of Cryptosporidium sp. isolates from human immunodeficiency virus-infected individuals in South India [46].

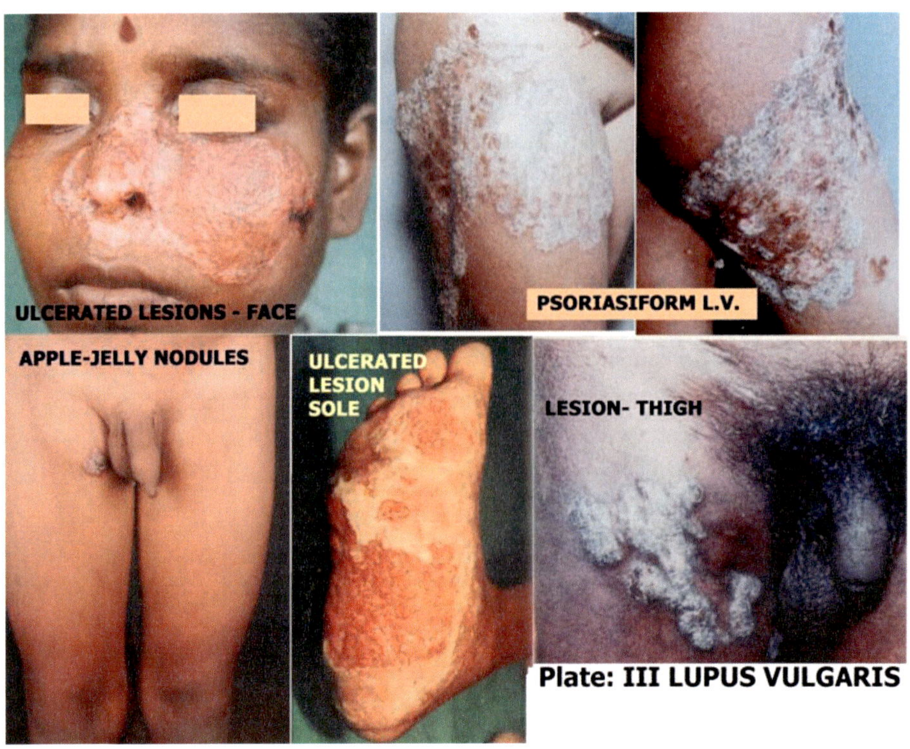

Plate: III LUPUS VULGARIS

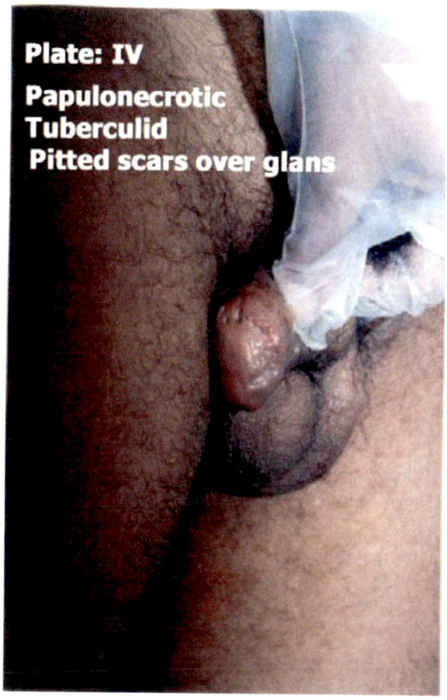

Plate: IV
Papulonecrotic Tuberculid
Pitted scars over glans

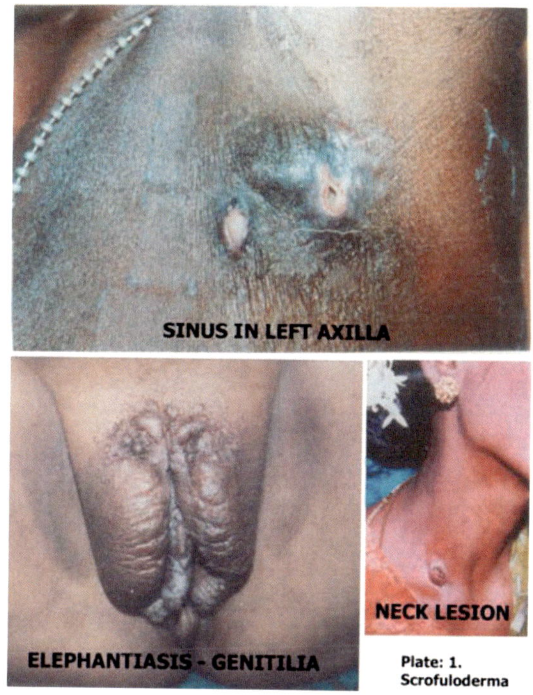

Plate: 1.
Scrofuloderma

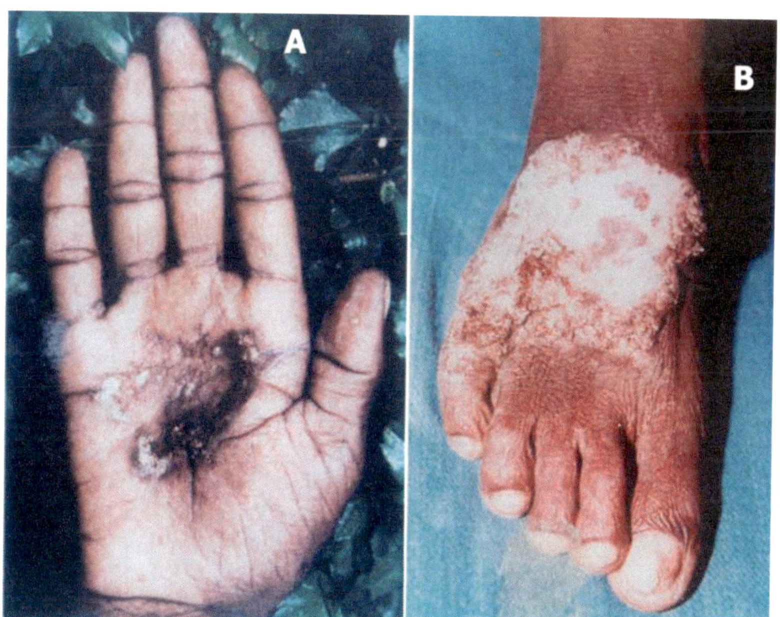

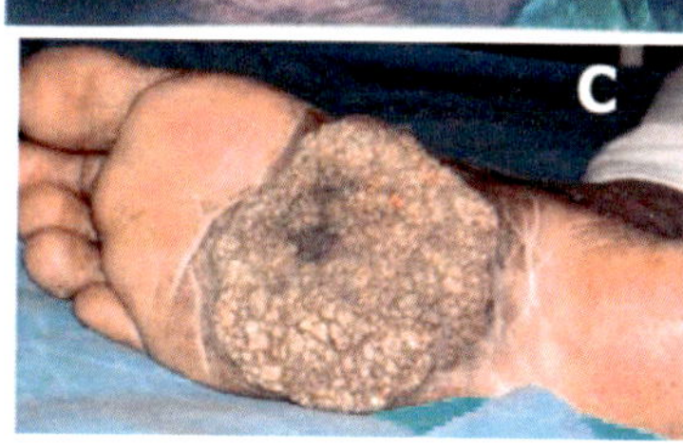

Plate: II
Tuberculosis Verrucosa Cutis
A. Lesion on Right Palm
B. Lesion on Dorsum of foot
C. Lesion on Sole

References

[1] Habibi B, Allain JP, Couroucé AM. Blood transfusion and acquired immunodeficiency syndrome (AIDS). *Rev Fr Transfus Immunohematol.* 1983 Nov;26(5):447-65.

[2] Batki SL. Drug abuse, psychiatric disorders, and AIDS. Dual and triple diagnosis. *West J Med.* 1990 May;152(5):547-52.

[3] Cohn JA. Virology, immunology, and natural history of HIV infection. *J Nurse Midwifery.* 1989 Sep-Oct;34(5):242-52.

[4] Lloyd A. HIV infection and AIDS. *P N G Med* J. 1996 Sep;39(3):174-80

[5] Horowitz HW, Telzak EE, Sepkowitz KA, Wormser GP. Human immunodeficiency virus infection, *Part I. Dis Mon.* 1998 Oct;44(10):545-606.

[6] Barnhart HX, Caldwell MB, Thomas P, Mascola L, Ortiz I, Hsu HW, Schulte J, Parrott R, Maldonado Y, Byers R.Natural history of human immunodeficiency virus disease in perinatally infected children: an analysis from the Pediatric Spectrum of Disease Project. *Pediatrics.* 1996 May;97(5):710-6.

[7] Purday BD, Plaisance KI.Infection with the human immunodeficiency virus: epidemiology, pathogenesis, transmission, diagnosis, and manifestations. *Am J Hosp Pharm.* 1989 Jun;46(6):1185-209.

[8] Pahwa S. Human immunodeficiency virus infection in children: nature of immunodeficiency, clinical spectrum and management. *Pediatr Infect Dis J.* 1988 May;7(5 Suppl):S61-71.

[9] Vial PA, Ferreccio C, Abarca K, Ortiz E, Noriega M, Pérez C, Labarca J, Torres M, Ferrés M, González C, Acuña G. Natural history of human immunodeficiency virus infection in a cohort of Chilean patients. *Rev Med Chil.* 1996 May;124(5):525-35.

[10] Prevention and treatment of tuberculosis among patients infected with human immunodeficiency virus: principles of therapy and revised recommendations. Centers for Disease Control and Prevention. *MMWR Recomm Rep.* 1998 Oct 30;47(RR-20):1-58.

[11] Lagnese M, Daar ES. Antiretroviral regimens for treatment-experienced patients with HIV-1 infection. *Expert Opin Pharmacother.* 2008 Apr;9(5):687-700.

[12] Lunzen J. Treatment of heavily antiretroviral-experienced HIV-infected patients. *AIDS Rev.* 2007 Oct-Dec;9(4):246-53.

[13] Hamers RL, Schuurman R, van Vugt M, Derdelinckx I, Rinke de Wit TF. AIDS treatment in Africa: the risk of antiretroviral resistance. Ned Tijdschr Geneeskd. 2007 Dec 1;151(48):2666-71.

[14] Mitsuya H, Maeda K, Das D, Ghosh AK. Development of protease inhibitors and the fight with drug-resistant HIV-1 variants. *Adv Pharmacol.* 2008;56:169-97.

[15] Martinez-Cajas JL, Wainberg MA. Antiretroviral therapy : optimal sequencing of therapy to avoid resistance. *Drugs.* 2008;68(1):43-72

[16] Menéndez-Arias L, Tözsér J. HIV-1 protease inhibitors: effects on HIV-2 replication and resistance. *Trends Pharmacol Sci.* 2008 Jan;29(1):42-9.

[17] Dunne M. Antiretroviral drug development: the challenge of cost and access. *AIDS.* 2007 Jul;21 Suppl 4:S73-9.

[18] Kolber MA. Development of drug resistance mutations in patients on highly active antiretroviral therapy: does competitive advantage drive evolution. *AIDS Rev.* 2007 Apr-Jun;9(2):68-74.

[19] Saliba G, Yeni P. Recent and future therapeutic advances in the management of HIV infection. *Pathol Biol (Paris).* 2006 Dec;54(10):545-50

[20] Shet A, Markowitz M.Transmitted multidrug resistant HIV-1: new and investigational therapeutic approaches. *Curr Opin Investig Drugs*. 2006 Aug;7(8):709-20.

[21] Sachdeva N, Sehgal S, Sud A, Datta U, Arora SK. Incidence of lamivudine resistance associated mutations in pol-gene of HIV-1 in patients from north India: a preliminary report. *Indian J Pathol Microbiol*. 2005 Jul;48(3):337-40.

[22] Pachamuthu B, Shanmugam S, Nagalingeswaran K, Solomon SS, Solomon S, Solomon S. HIV-1 drug resistance among untreated patients in India: Current status. *J Postgrad Med*. 2006 Jul-Sep;52(3):183-6.

[23] Saple DG, Vaidya SB, Vadrevu R, Pandey VP, Ramnani JP. Difficulties encountered with the use of antiretroviral drugs in India. *J HIV Ther*. 2002 Aug;7(3):56-8.

[24] Nagelkerke NJ, Jha P, de Vlas SJ, Korenromp EL, Moses S, Blanchard JF, Plummer FA. Modelling HIV/AIDS epidemics in Botswana and India: impact of interventions to prevent transmission. *Bull World Health Organ*. 2002;80(2):89-96.

[25] Kumarasamy N, Solomon S, Peters E, Amalraj RE, Purnima M, Ravikumar B, Yepthomi T, Thyagarajan SP. Antiretroviral drugs in the treatment of people living with human immunodeficiency virus: experience in a south Indian tertiary referral centre. *J Assoc Physicians India*. 2000 Apr;48(4):390-3.

[26] McMichael AJ. HIV vaccines. *Annu Rev Immunol*. 2006;24:227-55.

[27] Bennett DE. The requirement for surveillance of HIV drug resistance within antiretroviral rollout in the developing world. *Curr Opin Infect Dis*. 2006;19:607-14.

[28] Klumpp K, Mirzadegan T. Recent progress in the design of small molecule inhibitors of HIV RNase H. *Curr Pharm Des*. 2006;12:1909-22.

[29] Das K, Sarafianos SG, Clark AD Jr, Boyer PL, Hughes SH, Arnold E. Crystal Structures of Clinically Relevant Lys103Asn/Tyr181Cys Double Mutant HIV-1 Reverse Transcriptase in Complexes with ATP and Non-nucleoside Inhibitor HBY 097. *J Mol Biol*. 2007 Jan 5;365(1):77-89.

[30] Goldberg DL. Bonding. In: Goldberg DL, ed. *Chemistry*. Singapore: McGraw Hill, 1989; 95 -118.

[31] Arnold E, Das K, Ding J, Yadav PN, Hsiou Y, Boyer PL, Hughes SH. Targeting HIV reverse transcriptase for anti-AIDS drug design: structural and biological considerations for chemotherapeutic strategies. *Drug Des Discov*. 1996;13:29-47.

[32] De Clercq E. HIV inhibitors targeted at the reverse transcriptase. *AIDS Res Hum Retroviruses*. 1992;8:119-34.

[33] Abubakar I, Aliyu SH, Arumugam C, Usman NK, Hunter PR. Treatment of cryptosporidiosis in immunocompromised individuals: systematic review and meta-analysis. *Br J Clin Pharmacol*. 2007 Apr;63(4):387-93.

[34] Hung CC, Tsaihong JC, Lee YT, Deng HY, Hsiao WH, Chang SY, Chang SC, Su KE. Prevalence of intestinal infection due to Cryptosporidium species among Taiwanese patients with human immunodeficiency virus infection. *J Formos Med Assoc*. 2007 Jan;106(1):31-5.

[35] Abubakar I, Aliyu SH, Arumugam C, Hunter PR, Usman NK. Prevention and treatment of cryptosporidiosis in immunocompromised patients. *Cochrane Database Syst Rev*. 2007 Jan 24;(1):CD004932.

[36] Kasper LH, Buzoni-Gatel D. Some Opportunistic Parasitic Infections in AIDS: Candidiasis, Pneumocystosis, Cryptosporidiosis, Toxoplasmosis. *Parasitol Today*. 1998 Apr;14(4):150-6.

[37] Siński E. Resistance to intestinal opportunistic infections using Cryptosporidium sp. as an example. *Wiad Parazytol*. 2000;46(1):29-40.

[38] Lifson AR, Rhame FS, Belloso WH, Dragsted UB, El-Sadr WM, Gatell JM, Hoy JF, Krum EA, Nelson R, Pedersen C, Pett SL, Davey RT Jr. Reporting and evaluation of HIV-related clinical endpoints in two multicenter international clinical trials. *HIV Clin Trials*. 2006 May-Jun;7(3):125-41.

[39] Zardi EM, Picardi A, Afeltra A. Treatment of cryptosporidiosis in immunocompromised hosts. *Chemotherapy*. 2005 Jul;51(4):193-6.

[40] Mottet C, El Wafa AA, Cavassini M, D'Acremont V, Delarive J. Infectious diarrhea. *Rev Med Suisse*. 2005 Jan 19;1(3):209-10, 213-7.

[41] Joachim A. Is Cryptosporidium a zoonotic agent? *Wien Klin Wochenschr*. 2004;116 Suppl 4:2-6.

[42] Smith HV, Corcoran GD. New drugs and treatment for cryptosporidiosis. *Curr Opin Infect Dis*. 2004 Dec;17(6):557-64.

[43] Kaushik K, Khurana S, Wanchu A, Malla N. Evaluation of staining techniques, antigen detection and nested PCR for the diagnosis of cryptosporidiosis in HIV seropositive and seronegative patients. *Acta Trop*. 2008 Jul;107(1):1-7.

[44] Jayalakshmi J, Appalaraju B, Mahadevan K. Evaluation of an enzyme-linked immunoassay for the detection of Cryptosporidium antigen in fecal specimens of HIV/AIDS patients. *Indian J Pathol Microbiol*. 2008 Jan-Mar;51(1):137-8.

[45] Rao Ajjampur SS, Asirvatham JR, Muthusamy D, Gladstone BP, Abraham OC, Mathai D, Ward H, Wanke C, Kang G. Clinical features & risk factors associated with cryptosporidiosis in HIV infected adults in India. *Indian J Med Res*. 2007 Dec;126(6):553-7.

[46] Muthusamy D, Rao SS, Ramani S, Monica B, Banerjee I, Abraham OC, Mathai DC, Primrose B, Muliyil J, Wanke CA, Ward HD, Kang G. Multilocus genotyping of Cryptosporidium sp. isolates from human immunodeficiency virus-infected individuals in South India. *J Clin Microbiol*. 2006 Feb;44(2):632-4.

[47] Cruz ML, Cardoso CA, Saavedra MC, Santos ED, Melino T. Congenital toxoplasmosis infection in an infant born to an HIV-1-infected mother. *Braz J Infect Dis*. 2000 Dec;11(6):610-1.

[48] Machala L, Kodym P, Rozsypal H, Staňková M, Sedlácek D. Recommendation for diagnostics and therapy of toxoplasmosis in persons with HIV infection. *Klin Mikrobiol Infekc Lek*. 2007 Dec;13(6):248-52.

[49] Dedicoat M, Livesley N. Management of toxoplasmic encephalitis in HIV-infected adults--a review. *S Afr Med J*. 2008 Jan;98(1):31-2.

[50] Davaro RE, Thirumalai A. Life-threatening complications of HIV infection. *J Intensive Care Med*. 2007 Mar-Apr;22(2):73-81.

[51] Sokolska V, Knysz B, Czapiga E, Gasiorowski J, Sasiadek M, Gładysz A. The role of brain magnetic resonance studies in the diagnostics of central nervous system lesions in HIV-1 positive patients. Wiad Lek. 2006;59(11-12):805-13.

[52] Carme B, Demar-Pierre M. Toxoplasmosis in French Guiana. Atypical (neo-)tropical features of a cosmopolitan parasitosis. *Med Trop (Mars)*. 2006 Oct;66(5):495-503.

[53] Kasper LH, Buzoni-Gatel D. Some Opportunistic Parasitic Infections in AIDS: Candidiasis, Pneumocystosis, Cryptosporidiosis, Toxoplasmosis. *Parasitol Today*. 1998 Apr;14(4):150-6.

[54] Corr P. Imaging of neuro-AIDS. *J Psychosom Res*. 2006 Sep;61(3):295-9.

[55] Dedicoat M, Livesley N. Management of toxoplasmic encephalitis in HIV-infected adults (with an emphasis on resource-poor settings). *Cochrane Database Syst Rev.* 2006 Jul 19;3:CD005420

[56] Palanisamy M, Madhavan B, Balasundaram MB, Andavar R, Venkatapathy N. Outbreak of ocular toxoplasmosis in Coimbatore, India. *Indian J Ophthalmol.* 2006 Jun;54(2):129-31.

[57] Shivaprakash MR, Parija SC, Sujatha S. Serovalence of toxoplasmosis in HIV infected patients in Pondicherry. *J Commun Dis.* 2001 Sep;33(3):221-3.

Index

A

B

C

D

E

F

G

H

I

M

N

O

P

T

U

V